*Rush*ing
Woman's
Syndrome

Other books by Dr. Libby :

Accidentally Overweight (Hay House, 2016)

Exhausted to Energized (2015)

Published by Little Green Frog Publishing Ltd:

The Calorie Fallacy (2014)

Sweet Food Story (2014)

Beauty From the Inside Out (2013)

Real Food Kitchen (2013)

Real Food Chef (2012)

Women's Wellness Wisdom (2016)

Published by Pan Macmillan Australia:

The Energy Guide (2017)

*Rush*ing Woman's Syndrome

The Impact of a Never-Ending
To-Do List and How to Stay Healthy
in Today's Busy World

Dr. Libby Weaver

HAY HOUSE

Carlsbad, California • New York City
London • Sydney • New Delhi

Published in the United Kingdom by:
Hay House UK Ltd, The Sixth Floor, Watson House,
54 Baker Street, London W1U 7BU
Tel: +44 (0)20 3927 7290; www.hayhouse.co.uk

Published and distributed in the United States of America by:
Hay House LLC, PO Box 5100, Carlsbad, CA 92018-5100
Tel: (1) 760 431 7695 or (800) 654 5126; www.hayhouse.com

Published and distributed in India by:
Hay House Publishers (India) Pvt Ltd, Muskaan Complex, Plot No.3, B-2,
Vasant Kunj, New Delhi 110 070
Tel: (91) 11 4176 1620; www.hayhouse.co.in

Text © Dr. Libby Weaver, 2010, 2017

Previously published by Little Green Frog Publishing Ltd., 2011
(ISBN: 978-0-473-20403-7)

The information given in this book should not be treated as a substitute for
professional medical advice; always consult a medical practitioner. Any use of
information in this book is at the reader's discretion and risk. Neither the author nor
the publisher can be held responsible for any loss, claim or damage arising out of
the use, or misuse, of the suggestions made, the failure to take medical advice or
for any material on third-party websites.

A catalogue record for this book is available from the British Library.

Tradepaper ISBN: 978-1-4019-7815-0
E-book ISBN: 978-1-78180-897-9
Audiobook ISBN: 978-1-4019-9175-3

Interior images: 14, 49, 58, 88, 89, 107, 141, 150, 151
© Dr. Libby Weaver; 120 © masia8; all other images Shutterstock

10 9 8 7 6 5 4 3 2 1

Printed in the United States of America

This product uses responsibly sourced papers and/or recycled materials. For more
information, see www.hayhouse.com.

For Kate, with thanks.

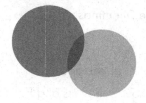

Contents

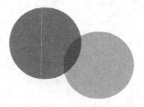

Acknowledgments

When I write, I hibernate and the work – brains and hearts – of numerous special humans allows me to do this. Thank you particularly to Kate, Maddy, Sarah, and Chris. I am very grateful to you.

Thank you to Amy, Julie, Sandy, and the team at Hay House UK for bringing this book to life in the northern hemisphere. I sincerely hope it makes a difference to women's health globally.

When I first caught a glimpse of what I have come to call 'Rushing Woman's Syndrome,' I wanted to assist women to take better care of their precious selves. I also want to take my hat off to them for all that they contribute to this world. You do all you do because of your deep care for people and the world. I simply want to help you to not do this at your own expense. Thank you amazing women everywhere.

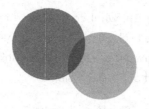

Introduction
Why Do Women Rush?

Rushing Woman's Syndrome evolved out of my observation of a shift in women's health and behavior over the past 18 years.

Never before in my work have I witnessed so many females in such an intense rush to do everything and be all things to all people. Never before have I seen the extent of reproductive system problems that I now see. Women are wired. Many of them are tired too. Tired yet wired. And this relentless urgency, this perception that there is not enough time combined with a never-ending to-do list, is having significant health consequences for many women.

The perceived need to rush, whether we show it on the outside or keep it under wraps, is changing women's health in a detrimental way. Sex hormone-based health issues, such as polycystic ovarian syndrome (PCOS), endometriosis, infertility, and debilitating menopause symptoms, not to mention exhaustion, have never been greater, while the role of stress is undeniable when you look at both our body's chemistry and the scientific research.

Imbalanced hormones, depleted adrenal glands from long-term overproduction of stress hormones, sluggish thyroid glands, and the impact of all of this on our health, as well as the people around us, concerns me greatly. Yet what concerns me just as much is 'why' we do it. Why do we think and behave in ways that are leading to this significant, downward spiral in our health? The answer lies in our biochemistry and our belief systems.

Once you understand what is really going on, you will see that the swing between rushing and not rushing is driven by our beliefs, and our behavior is the expression of those beliefs. Unless we question the beliefs upon which our actions are based, the actions will likely continue.

Regardless of the circumstances, when you feel or perceive that your life is challenging, no matter how big or how small those challenges, they have an impact. What you perceive is then hormonally generated by your biochemistry.

For many, the body cannot keep up with the rate of change the world now asks of it and so it is imperative that we take steps to create periods of downtime: days, weeks, or months when we can truly rest. Just as we can't go without sleep for too long, the psyche cannot push on for too long without getting some quality rest. If it does, science and our intuition both tell us, there will be consequences.

What's changed?

All species on the planet evolve every time they reproduce. The idea is that each new generation will be better equipped to cope with the prevailing conditions, the environment. Our challenge is that our surroundings are changing at a rate never before witnessed in human evolution.

Science tells us that human beings have been on the Earth for 150,000–200,000 years. Our ancient ancestors were nomadic and lived off the land, and ate what surrounded them, as they moved. As hunters and gatherers, the weather conditions, climate, and seasons influenced our daily movement patterns and what we ate. Daily tasks revolved around what needed to be done to stay alive and we ate food as it came from nature – primarily green leaves and other more concentrated foods, such as meat, fish, fruits, nuts and seeds only as the opportunity arose.

It was only 7,500–10,000 years ago that our ancestors began to stay in one place for longer periods of time. The birth of agriculture allowed us to grow crops, and for the first time in human history we consumed the milk of other animals. While our patterns of living and eating were still based on nature's seasonal rhythms, and at the mercy of what could be completed within daylight hours, we no longer had to chase our food down and had a relatively consistent supply of food.

During this period, change continued at a steady and gradual pace and the chemistry of our body was able to keep up. With the Industrial Revolution in the 19th century, however, change began to quicken as processes were mechanized and we began leaving the land and flocking to cities to work, creating an increased reliance on agriculture to feed everyone. A day's work also required less movement, and standards of living became very much aligned to where we lived and how much we earned.

The past three decades have seen a faster, more dramatic change. We've welcomed the Internet into our lives in an increasingly big way and seen the invention of cell phones. Prior to this advance in technology nobody could reach us as we drove to and from work, or when we were taking the kids to school or shopping. Today our cell phones ring, ping and vibrate incessantly to inform us of the arrival of e-mails, calls, and social media notifications – at all times of the day and night. Unless we choose to have boundaries around when we are contactable, we are essentially on call 24/7.

So many people use every single spare moment to check for texts and e-mails, or catch up on the latest update from their favorite social media portal – including while waiting at traffic lights. It wasn't long ago that, while we were waiting for the lights to turn green, we only had our surroundings to observe or our own thoughts to contemplate, or a song to groove to on the radio. There was naturally, without effort, more soul food and downtime in our lives, and less temptation to fill every spare moment with something 'productive.'

We've also seen an enormous change in the way we eat. Very few of us now live off the land in the West, and many of us choose to get our nourishment from non-food ingredients out of packs because we're in such a rush – and the quicker the better. For many, if food isn't convenient it is simply not on the menu. You don't need me to tell you that this kind of eating comes at a cost. You'd have had to have your head buried in the sand not to know we need to be eating a diet of mostly fresh foods and that most of us need to eat way more vegetables than we currently do.

But more often than not it is our beliefs, rather than a lack of education, that drives us to make poor food choices. While in some cases further education about food, nutrition, lifestyle choices, and wellbeing can be immensely beneficial, from where I'm sitting, inspiration and unraveling your beliefs about your wellbeing is just as important. That uplifting feeling of wanting to take good care of yourself and believing that you are worth it.

Out of sync with nature

I observe people, particularly at airports, as they step onto moving walkways and stop, rather than continuing to walk. They're exhausted and take every opportunity to rest. Contraptions like moving walkways were designed to help us get places faster, yet some of these things are not supportive to our health, as they stop us from moving. We have elevators, escalators, moving walkways, and transportation so we no longer have to climb stairs or walk long distances. Forget harvesting our own food or chasing it down with a spear, we don't even have to go to the store if we don't want to. We can buy our food online and have someone deliver it. There is no judgment here. Merely a tip of the iceberg of observation, as to how quickly and significantly the world we live in has changed.

We are guinea pigs in so many areas, often without even realizing it. Never before has the population been exposed to pesticides for their entire lifetimes or had a device that is known to emit radiation so close to our brains on a regular basis. No population has ever consumed artificial sweeteners, colors, preservatives, and trans fats through the entirety of a lifetime. I have every finger and toe crossed, and even my eyes, hoping that all of these things are safe. My instincts tell me that hope and reality don't match.

While the world around us has changed rapidly, at a cellular level our bodies are basically the same as our predecessors'. While every generation evolves ever so slightly to be better equipped to inhabit its environment, the rate of evolution is nothing compared to the change of pace in our world. Our conscious, thinking minds may have developed the capacity to keep up so that we can e-mail while talking on our cell phone, as we recall we need to order a cake for our child's birthday (notice I inferred buy rather than bake), but our biochemistry remains much the same as it was 150,000 years ago.

Just as importantly our subconscious mind, which is one million more times more powerful than our conscious mind, is still relatively the same. You cannot access your subconscious with your thoughts, but it controls the biological functions and systems in the body from your heartbeat to your hair growth, and it knows how to heal a cut without you having to tell it to do so. I do not believe that the human nervous system is able to meet the demands that this time in human history asks of it.

We are asking the body to go places it has never ever been before. Never before have we had a communication system that means we are always connected so that we are simultaneously distracted and overstimulated. Or been 'too busy' to prepare our own food. Or do any exercise whatsoever. What we are yet to truly understand in the West is that urgency, and the pace that we feel required to live at, is a disaster for our health, particularly for our nervous and our reproductive systems.

We have become so far removed from our origins that many people believe it's a luxury or a fad to eat seasonal produce, to turn off their cell phone at night, take their shoes off to feel the earth beneath their bare feet, not respond to e-mails within three minutes of receiving them, and take a day of rest or leisure each week. And yes, that does mean a day where even e-mails and social feeds go unchecked.

We seem to have fallen out of sync with the guiding light of nature, not just regarding our food but our whole way of living. What if Mother Nature does know best? It wasn't all that long ago that we treated colds with garlic and lemon. Now, we take a pill and race on because we believe we can't afford the time off work. We go on vacation for a week and do three weeks' worth of work the week before we leave, just to get the work done, and then have to catch up on a week's worth of e-mails and work when we get back.

Personal cost

Take a step back and it sounds like we've lost our minds, doesn't it? Essentially, it takes awareness and a commitment to live another way, a way that is more supportive of health on every level. Nutrients keep the body alive and with whole foods we are better nourished. With more free time, our relationships are nurtured, and we tend to be happier and kinder to both ourselves and those around us.

You might notice the impact of the rush on your external world – perhaps in the lack of downtime or on your closest relationships – yet when you ask your glands and organs – your liver, your gallbladder, your kidneys, your adrenals, your thyroid, your ovaries, your uterus, your brain, and your digestive system – to cope with your rush, you may not even realize what undue stress you're putting them under. These are some of the consequences to this superfast pace of living, and this book is partly born out of my observations and reflections, as well as the science behind what modern life is requiring of and doing to women.

Our bodies are not wired to cope with constant pressure, perceived or real, nor are we equipped long-term to eat poor-quality food and lead sedentary lifestyles, strapped to technology, plugged in and switched on. As I said, this is the tip of a partially inglorious but incredibly fascinating iceberg, and I hope this book will help you become aware of what the rush is doing to your body and why you may have become caught up in it. Becoming aware of how and why you rush is the first step to altering this way of living and while some of the information is likely new for you, you'll also discover reminders of what you already know.

In writing this book I have used numerous examples and real-life stories of rushing women of all ages and walks of life. A common scenario is one of a working heterosexual mother. However, there are a multitude of other scenarios involving work, life, sexual preferences, relationship status, or socioeconomic situations that may or may not include children. I tell stories to help get the message across and I just wanted you to know that sometimes I generalize and recount what I hear most often... which is just one side of the story, after all.

Reflect and Action

You'll find opportunities throughout this book to reflect and take action to shift from a rushed state to a calmer one, as well as an entire section dedicated to helping you support your physical body and improve your mental wellbeing. You may find it helpful to keep a pen and paper or your journal handy to take a note of any answers, ideas or solutions that arise while reading.

I am aware that men suffer from the rush too. I witness it every day. But the male psyche is somewhat different from the female so I have chosen to concentrate on women for this book. That is certainly not because I don't care about our men nor do I believe that their health is not being compromised by pressure and stress. I simply want to explore thoroughly why women are in a hurry more than ever before, the consequences of it, and of course offer insights and strategies that have the potential to foster change.

If you have read my first book, *Accidentally Overweight*, you may know of the effects of stress on your waistline, as it explores what has to happen for the body to get the message to burn or store fat. But this book is also about modern lifestyles and the impact of stress on all our body systems, as well as our relationships, and I sincerely hope you find plenty of new and helpful advice in the following chapters.

There will only ever be 24 hours in a day. And how you spend your time is entirely your choice. Your perception of how you need to be and what you need to do in a day is influenced by both your biochemistry and your beliefs. And you are about to gain some brand-new insights into both. Come with me on this journey and take your understanding of your health to a whole new level, and utilize the strategies and rituals offered here to change your health future.

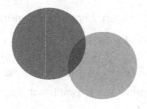

Chapter 1

Too Busy to Stop

What Is Rushing Woman's Syndrome?

Rushing Woman's Syndrome (RWS) describes the biochemical effects of always being in a hurry and the health consequences that urgency elicits. It is not a medical diagnosis, but rather a title I gave to the myriad changes I was witnessing in women's health, and to help my patients better understand their own health picture.

Imagine if you will RWS in action.

It doesn't seem to matter whether she has two things to do or 200, she is often in a pressing rush to do it all. Wound up like a spring, she runs herself ragged in a daily battle to keep up. There is always so much to do, and she very rarely feels like she wins, is in control, or gets on top of things. In fact her deep desire to control even the smaller details of life can leave her feeling out of control, even of herself.

Overwhelmed, at times she feels like she can't cope, whether she admits it out loud or keeps it all inside, adding to her wound-up, knotted stomach. She is fortunate if her sex hormones are balanced. Most women with RWS suffer terribly with their periods or don't bleed regularly, and women who go into menopause in this state usually find it debilitating.

There is a subgroup of RWS that I lovingly call the 'thyroid types.' These women cherish their coffee to the point that they feel they cannot live without it. They tell me that it clears the fog in their brain, gives them a tiny amount of energy (which is better than none), and that it keeps their bowels moving. They almost always tell me that coffee makes them happy. Thyroid types are less wired than others. It takes a lot of caffeine to amp them up. Thyroids are mostly tired. Beyond tired actually. The fatigue is in their bones, whereas the majority of rushing women are wired and typically get very weary in the late afternoon to early evening, but if they stay up after 10 p.m. they often get a second wind and it is then very hard to go to sleep until 1 or 2 a.m.

The following is a checklist to help you identify if you are indeed a rushing woman:

- Loves coffee to the point that she feels deprived if she cannot get her daily fix, and says she needs it for energy, to help her brain function, or to make her bowels move.

- Answers 'so busy' or 'stressed' when you ask her how she is.

- Experiences stress hormones, adrenalin (also known as epinephrine), and cortisol, pumping through her veins more often than she does not.

- Has low progesterone (see Chapter 2, page 28).

- Experiences challenges with menstruation, which might involve heavy, clotty, painful, and/or irregular periods, premenstrual stress (PMS), polycystic ovarian syndrome (PCOS), or a debilitating menopause.

- Tends to crave sugar, particularly mid-afternoon or close to menstruation.

- Often feels overwhelmed.

- Has a poor short-term memory.

- Feels like there are never enough hours in the day.

- Overreacts easily, even if she doesn't display it outwardly.

- Often feels tired but wired.

- May have a thyroid gland that bounces between an underactive and overactive tendency.

- Can't sit down, as she feels guilty unless she is beyond tired – then she will sit but still feels guilty.

- Does not get enough sleep and sometimes cannot sleep restoratively.

- Compromises sleep to get jobs done late at night.

- Is irritable or, as I prefer to say, 'gritty.'

- Wants to speed when she drives, whether she needs to or not, wonders why everyone else drives so slowly – whether they do or not.

- Has no solitude, no time for self, and will tell you that's selfish or a luxury she could never have.

- Has a to-do list that is never completed, and this bothers her.

- Feels a sense of panic easily.

- Experiences frequent digestive system problems, such as bloating or irritable bowel syndrome (IBS).

- Is so exhausted, particularly in the afternoon, a time when she is also more likely to feel like she cannot cope with her life – sugar, caffeine or alcohol feel like the only options at this time.

- Regularly fails to notice the special moments of life, as it feels mostly chaotic.

- Laughs less than she used to.

- Finds it difficult to relax without alcohol.

- Has a mental fuzziness/haze/brain fog that she only notices if she has a random day when her head feels clear.

- Beats herself up for not being a good enough wife/mother/ friend.

- Is constantly looking for more ways to feel love or be praised, whether she can see this or not.

- Feels anxious without her cell phone and catches herself constantly pushing the refresh screen button, in case she misses an important message or text – and for this reason checks her e-mail at traffic lights and late at night, and takes her phone to the bathroom.

- Goes on vacation only to spend the majority of the time thinking about unwinding, yet never actually resting, and it simply becomes an extension of her usual life.

- Tends to return from a break feeling even more exhausted than before she left.

- Takes short and shallow breaths and can often become breathless; may sigh frequently.

- Low appetite or, on the contrary, feels as though she could eat her arm off, particularly at night.

- Tends to blame others for adding to her workload or 'stressing her out' – when at least some of the stress is due to internal pressures.

- Goes to guilt as a common emotional pattern.

- Doesn't usually ask for help.

- Can't say no easily and if she does... feels guilty!

Reflect

How many of the above statements do you relate to? To have a bit of fun with this, count the number of statements you relate to and explore your level of rushing using the scale below!

0 = This book is not for you. But read on, as it will more than likely relate to some of your friends.

1–7 = You are not a rushing woman but may find this book helpful in identifying the areas of your endocrine system that may need some extra support. For example, if you experience PMS, apply the strategies suggested for that particular condition.

7–15 = You are well on your way to becoming a rushing woman. Apply the strategies suggested to support your physical and emotional health, and get your score down and level of wellbeing up.

15 or above = Hello rushing woman. It is delightful to meet you and to be able to assist you to come down from the stress mountain.

Physical health of a rushing woman

There are a number of body systems involved in the rush. They include the:

- Nervous system

- Endocrine system, which includes the adrenal glands, ovaries, thyroid gland and pituitary gland

- Digestive system

Any or all of the above systems may be affected by a hurried lifestyle. When you address just one of these systems, you might feel somewhat better. However, if the mad rush continues, your overall health is likely to continue to suffer and potentially decline. Helping you sort out your biochemistry is a big part of what this book is intended to do. In the next few chapters, you will learn not only how to identify which of your systems needs attention and particular care, but also what to do about it.

When your biochemistry is out of whack – for example, your sex hormones – it can be very difficult to change how you feel. You may suffer from a tendency to get stuck in overwhelm, have frequent meltdowns, burst with angry explosions, or all of the above. Your body constantly receives messages from the environment and from itself about the chemicals (hormones) it needs to make and sorting these out can go a long way toward helping you slow down and not feel like everything had to be done yesterday.

Take a deep breath and come with me on a journey of hormones, thoughts and perceptions, energy and vitality.

The emotional health of a rushing woman

There is far more to being a rushing woman than simply your hormones being out of balance. You haven't always been like this. You certainly weren't born in this state. The rush is learned.

You can most likely recall a time in your life when everything somehow seemed simpler, and you may find yourself craving this feeling again. Yet when you look at how you might alter your current life, you often feel helpless to change anything because things seem intertwined and therefore complicated. For example, 'If I go part-time so I can spend more time with the children, we can't make the mortgage repayments and pay our bills. I'm exhausted and yet I'm aware my husband is under just as much pressure. And if I reduce my paid work he will feel even more financial pressure and I worry about his health, for his sake and of course the children's, and so it is just easier if I keep doing everything.'

Do you know how many times I've heard versions of this sentiment? Thousands. And I have to admit that there is a part of me that wants to tell people to sell their house, buy something cheaper, spend less, want less from a material perspective – because I am yet to experience a house that comes even close to outweighing the importance of human health. No house is worth it. Sure this is only one scenario but it demonstrates how our desire to take better care of ourselves can sometimes feel like an impossible dream. But every knotted piece of string has two ends. Find one of them and ask for help to unravel it, if you cannot see the way forward yourself.

The present pace of life has catapulted us into a new realm with unique pressures and an unprecedented intensity. Our mothers and grandmothers didn't have cell phones and e-mails and more office work to attend to after the kitchen was cleaned and the washing and ironing put away – times have changed. Our mothers had their own way of dealing with the pressures they felt. They may have spent money, if they had it, or eaten too much. Some of them drank too much alcohol and some might have been outwardly content yet very worried on the inside. Most females have always been scared about 'getting into trouble' or 'letting others down.' It is just that now, from the push, push, push and the rush, rush, rush of technology, a significant feminine emotional pattern is emerging. And our nervous systems, our reproductive systems, and our digestive systems are suffering, as a result of it. What is it? What is this emotional pattern I'm claiming has been around for longer than the rush – that the rush has brought closer to the surface, more out into the open – for a health professional like me to observe?

The why

This is a big bold statement: Rushing Woman's Syndrome comes from our relentless pursuit to never feel rejected.

Our deepest need to never feel rejected establishes itself when we are young children. It might have arisen due to a look on your mother's face, the way your parents might have cut you off with their impatient tones when you had something important to say, or your father's odd behavior when he'd had too much to drink. From any, or all, of these scenarios, or another that is particular to you, you created a meaning that your parents didn't love you and that you had to do something – rather than just be you – to be loved. And you've spent the rest of your life, on some level, doing absolutely everything you can to never, ever feel that way – shut out, unloved, ostracized, abandoned, neglected – again. So you please people. Anyone and everyone. You can't sleep if you are worried you've upset someone. If you particularly, desperately have to please your intimate partner (and if he is male or she has a masculine essence), you have a stronger connection to avoiding rejection set up by interactions with your father than your mother. Whereas if your partner comes way down your list in your 'urgency to please' behavior, your fear of rejection probably stems from your feminine role model, most often your mother.

Many rushing women despise conflict. They will often do anything to avoid it – including 'alter the truth' while their motto is 'keep the peace.' I am stunned by the number of women, and women who earn their own money, who lie to their husbands about what they spend. I regularly hear tales from women who have gone shopping and bought a pair of boots and a handbag (for example), which they'd been eyeing for ages, and then scuffed them both so that husbands wouldn't notice that they were new and ask what they cost. Another friend used a marker to change the price on the ticket of a top she had bought so it looked like the top was discounted. When I asked what would happen if he found out that she'd paid full price for the top, she said, 'I'd get into trouble' – this from a grown woman who works hard running her own business.

> **Reflect**
>
> Start to reflect on your own behaviors. You may not change the price of things but there are potentially other things you do to keep the peace. Yet consider, that there is no peace when you have to keep the peace.

Our adrenal glands, the place in the body where our stress hormones are made, are often in overdrive, as a result of stress – both physical and emotional. Physical stress comes from a low-nutrient diet, lack of sleep, too many processed foods and drinks, which make it hard for the liver to work optimally and efficiently – and emotional stress from, for example, the relentless urgency to please and avoid rejection. And when stress hormones are consistently elevated, our sex hormone balance is massively disrupted; we will explore these concepts in detail later in the book. All you need to know right now is that you can unravel this. It is a physical, emotional, and spiritual journey that can be, at times, challenging and confronting, yet utterly magnificent, enlightening, and, ultimately, one that reminds you that the peace you seek is within you.

There is a concept in emergency medicine called triage, where patients are assigned a degree of urgency based on how quickly their wounds need treatment. This is what women do all day long. Our daily existence can involve the constant assessment of who needs our attention the most: children, husband, work, best friend, mother, kind neighbor, not-so-kind neighbor, unwell friend, overflowing laundry basket... We tend to leave ourselves off this list, yet if I were to ask the majority of women if they believe they have omitted themselves because they are selfless, most reply with an emphatic 'No! I simply don't have time.' If we don't have time for ourselves, soon we'll have nothing left to give.

Peace is always present

It is easy to get caught up in a story you tell yourself about how hard/busy/tough/never-ending/overwhelming your life is. And it is so easy to blame the people around you. You cannot change them. You can only change yourself. And if you pause and focus on this precise moment, there is nothing but peace and beauty, and that can permeate your entire existence if that is what you want. It is always there, always available, waiting for you to notice.

I witnessed a friend recently throw away an opportunity to be present when I commented on how precious her three children's clothes looked, hanging on the staircase railing, all pressed and tiny and ready for school the next day. And their little shoes lined up beneath each outfit. When I commented to my friend on what a sweet sight it was, she (bless her in her exhaustion) rolled her eyes and said it is Groundhog Day to her. In an instant she saw what she had done – washed over a moment in time, missed soaking up the soul-nourishing sight at the bottom of the stairs, as her mind had jumped ahead to what tomorrow would bring – another morning of feeling beyond exhausted and of chaos and demands on her time and energy.

The beauty of life is there to behold if we can BE in the moment, rather than always being ahead of it. Yes, we have to plan and organize, of course we do. But my goodness the feelings of stress are so much less when we have moments of noticing and soaking up the immense beauty around us. And the stress is so much less if we invest in ourselves, whatever that looks like for you. Going to your local café and reading a magazine, sitting outside your home and letting the sun warm your back, with only the birds to keep you company, starting the day with qi gong (also known as chi kung) and a walk. Part of what I will encourage you to do in the following chapters is to shift your perception from feeling there is never enough time to creating spaciousness in your life. From shifting your perception from 'I have to do all of this' to 'wow, I get to do all of this.'

But before we get into how to shift from rush to calm, I'd like to share one final point for you to consider about what all this rushing might be doing to you.

I spoke at a lunch with a friend of mine who is a psychologist. He asked the audience of women to describe what romance meant to them. The majority of the women in the room responded with comments such as 'when he vacuums the floor' and 'when he takes the garbage out without being asked.' Very few responded with what they may have been more likely to say at the beginning of a courtship such as 'calling me outside to share a sunset,' 'a bunch of flowers for no reason,' and 'my husband's face lighting up when he sees me.' And what struck me, with the majority of comments being focused on helping around the house, was how time-poor women perceive themselves to be. If taking out the garbage has become romance, you definitely feel that you have too much on your plate to handle!

There would not have been a woman in the room who married her husband for his vacuuming skills! Yet this is what many women have come to perceive as romance – help. I am not denying for one second that receiving help makes an enormous difference to how we feel and that teamwork in a marriage is vital. What I am saying is that when taking out the garbage has become how you want romance demonstrated to you, you are overwhelmed with your to-do list, and it is time for things to change or for a new perspective.

Not so long ago, women began doing what had historically been their father's jobs, while many maintained their mother's responsibilities. What has transpired for so many women is a frantic double shift, of work day and night, with very little rest. We are capable, of course we are. Yet what I want you to grasp is that this is the very first time in all of human history that we have asked our body to live in this way. And for too many women their health is suffering as a result, for we have not yet evolved to be able to cope with living this way.

Women are carrying around copious amounts of information that won't seem to leave them alone. To paraphrase the brilliant Allison Pearson, the inside of a woman's head is akin to an international airport, as her mind races along at a million miles an hour thinking about everything from reading programs and fixing the car to whether she's changed her mind about that guy she met last week... *must text him*, and the six reports that were due to the client an hour ago.

My friend Amanda calls them 'first-world problems.' All this information just circles around in our heads, awaiting further instruction from air traffic control. If women didn't bring all that they do safely in to land, the whole world would fall apart. Instead, the health of women is coming undone in a way that is preventable.

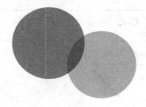

Chapter 2
Tired But Wired

The Impact of Rush on Your Nervous System

When it comes to your health and your degree of calm, one body system stands out above all others – the nervous system.

Comprised of various body parts – including your brain, your spinal cord, and the nerves that connect your brain to every organ of your body – there are several components to the nervous system, two of which are:

- Central nervous system (CNS)

- Autonomic nervous system (ANS), which has two branches: sympathetic nervous system (SNS) and parasympathetic nervous system (PNS)

Rather than worrying about remembering all of these long-winded names, just know that the SNS drives the fight-or-flight response, while the PNS promotes rest and digest, also known as the rest-and-repair response. This is diagrammatically represented in figure 1 on the following page.

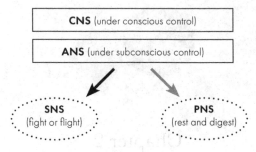

Figure 1: Parts of the nervous system
The CNS and ANS are controlled separately, while the
SNS and the PNS are branches of the ANS.

The CNS is governed by your conscious mind and you control it with your thoughts. For example, if you want to write, you choose to pick up a pen and write. If you choose to walk, you control the direction and the pace. You choose it. Your ANS, however, is controlled by your subconscious mind. In other words you are unable to access it with your thoughts. Your ANS controls all the functions of your body: heart rate, cell renewal, digestion, etc.

You cannot suddenly wake up and tell the ANS to grow hair down to your waist – it doesn't work like that. Your hair will grow to your waist (if that's what you want!) in its own sweet time. You have no say in it. It is the ANS that is so enormously affected by rushing, and you are also enormously affected by the way your ANS responds to what you may not even realize you think about or perceive.

Before we proceed any further in understanding the role of the nervous system in your health, I first want to share with you the symptoms your body might present with, if the nervous system is indeed a challenge for you, and a body system that needs support.

- You regularly feel stressed or on red alert.

- No matter how carefully you count calories and exercise, your body shape and size is a mystery to you.

- You crave sugars and/or starches (carbohydrates).

- You love coffee, energy drinks; anything that contains caffeine, although sometimes you notice they make your heart race.

- You startle (jump) easily.

- You often don't sleep well.

- You don't wake up restored or with good energy.

- If you don't go to sleep by 10 p.m., you get a second wind and end up staying awake until at least 1 a.m. (this can be a classic sign of adrenal fatigue, see Chapter 4, page 56).

- You regularly feel tired but wired.

- You are a worrier or a drama queen.

- You feel anxious easily.

- Your breathing tends to be shallow and quite fast.

- You experience 'air hunger' (and other causes have been ruled out).

- You struggle to say 'no.'

- You laugh less than you used to.

- Everything seems urgent.

- You feel like there aren't enough hours in the day.

The nervous system and body fat

Let's start by looking at the role that the nervous system plays in using fat as its fuel and weight gain, as this is often a source of frustration and stress for many women and makes them hurry around even more. So yes, rushing around doesn't just negatively affect wellbeing but also causes many women to store unnecessary fat.

In any given moment the human body is making a decision about which fuel to use based on the information it receives. The only two fuels for the human body are glucose ('sugar') and fat. You don't use protein for fuel. The body breaks protein down into amino acids, which are then converted into glucose so the body can use that glucose as fuel (energy). The body requires energy for everything it does, from walking to sleeping, from laughing to blinking; it all requires fuel.

Adrenalin, one of the stress hormones, communicates to every cell of your body that your life is in danger and it prepares you to fight or flee. However, you may be making adrenalin simply because you have to make a phone call that you'd rather not make or perhaps because you've gulped down three cups of coffee already. The stress for most people in the West today is psychological rather than physical.

The branch of the nervous system that is activated by stress of any type is the sympathetic nervous system (SNS), which has an intimate relationship with adrenalin. If the body perceives that it needs to escape from impending danger, whether your thinking mind is telling you so or not, you need a fast-burning fuel available to you to do that. Your body thinks it has to get out of there and get out of there fast!

Remember the body's only choice is to burn either sugar or fat, and in a fight-or-flight scenario, it will choose sugar every time. The body is all about survival and because it perceives a threat (due to adrenalin production) it doesn't feel 'safe' enough to use fat as its fuel in this fight-or-flight state because fat offers us a steady, slow-release form of energy. We can burn fat effectively in a PNS-dominant state because the body perceives it is safe. Yet, the PNS can never be the dominant arm of the ANS, it can never steer the ship, while the body perceives there may be a threat to your life.

Glucose is stored in our muscles and liver in a form called glycogen, and these stores are mobilized whenever the body gets the message that it needs energy to fight or flee. If there is not enough to fuel our escape left in our blood from our last meal then it will use glycogen from our muscles, and this can, over time, impact the function and appearance of our muscles, including the onset of cellulite, particularly at the top of your legs.

I believe that one of the most enormous health challenges of modern times is that the body can constantly be on the receiving end of the fight-or-flight message. There are so many factors, internal and external, that can drive this response within us, which we'll explore shortly, but first let's explore why most diets don't work.

Reflect

When could you actively choose not to go there, not to get caught up in the rush, and take steps to allow your nervous system to have some balance?

Most people believe that you need to lose weight in order to be healthy but in my work, what I have seen is the opposite – you need to be healthy before you can lose weight. I have worked with many people who subsist on very few calories and exercise rampantly, but never seem to be able to drop their weight.

How else can we approach this? And how does this lifestyle create what I, with kindness, refer to as Rushing Woman's Syndrome? For some, this is at the heart of them becoming what I lovingly titled my first book, *Accidentally Overweight*. Don't get me wrong, some rushing women are slim. But their nervous systems are usually a wreck, and a nervous system imbalance takes a significant toll on our health, hormones and usually our relationships. For example, you may not understand why you now react with intensity to situations you once spoke about calmly, such as when someone leaves the butter out.

The nervous system and weight loss

In general, the SNS and the PNS work in sync but with opposite functions. The primary role of the SNS, as you now know, is to keep us safe. So when we are stressed, it raises our heart rate, increases our respiratory rate, releases cortisol, and shunts blood away from the digestive tract to the muscles to give us the energy to fight or flee.

If we are experiencing mental or emotional stress, or our organ systems are unhealthy, and therefore stressed, this also activates the SNS, so we can easily find ourselves with additional load in this system. By its very nature, the SNS is catabolic – overstimulation of the SNS increases the secretion of cortisol, which breaks down muscle tissues.

What you might not have considered is that high-intensity exercise is also sympathetic in nature – it increases our heart rate, respiration and body temperature, and as a result cortisol is released into the blood, which signals to the body to store fat and interrupts our sex hormone production.

Once the 'threat' is dealt with (keeping in mind that if we're talking about mental or emotional stress, it might never be dealt with) the PNS kicks in to slow our heart rate and respiration, move blood back to the digestive tract so we're able to digest our food and be well nourished, works on repairing any tissues that have been damaged in our 'battle,' and allows libido to be restored. Your survival instinct can't have you thinking about sex when your body believes that your life is being threatened!

If we go to bed early enough, the PNS is able to do its wonderful work overnight. If we're night owls, cortisol naturally starts to rise at around 2 a.m. and the less sleep we get before that time, the less time our PNS has to do its work. The SNS and the PNS are designed to balance each other, and high-intensity exercise will lead to fat loss in those people who have a well-balanced nervous system since muscle tissue is built in the parasympathetic rest time between workouts.

Those who find they are unable to lose fat through regular high-intensity exercise are likely have a dominant SNS and, consequently, an inhibited PNS. In situations like this where there is too much systemic 'stress' coming from somewhere, high-intensity exercise exacerbates the nervous system imbalance by adding to the individual's sympathetic load and is counterproductive. This is one of the reasons why the 'calorie in versus calorie out' theory is defunct when it comes to weight loss. If 'burning' more calories is yet to solve your body-fat challenge, it's not going to start doing so until your other body systems are working optimally.

Even without considering anxiety – something that many people experience in our world today from relationship challenges, financial stress, concerns about health, a fixation on weight, and the consequences of a poor diet – your SNS may be in overload. And so many people won't even mention being stressed or anxious! Alarmingly, not living this way is becoming the exception.

What's more, reducing the sympathetic load is essential to weight loss if the SNS is dominant.

Action

Effective exercise for SNS-dominant people is what I call the more 'yin' (gentle, feminine, as opposed to 'yang,' masculine, go go go) forms of exercise, such as tai chi, qi gong, restorative yoga or any exercise that is done slowly, while being conscious of the breath. These types of exercise significantly assist in increasing PNS activity, which helps balance the ANS. Once the nervous system is better balanced, body fat is readily burned.

Sympathetic nervous system (SNS) dominance

The majority of women I see in my practice and at my women's health weekends, and even those I meet on the street, are SNS dominant. Their perception of what they have to do in a day is overwhelming to them. They have usually elevated their adrenalin production and pushed themselves further into SNS dominance with caffeine in the morning as well. Even the calmest, most grounded woman will be fizzing, on the inside at least, with a few coffees under her belt. For some, even one caffeinated beverage is enough to amp them up so significantly that they overreact to the smallest thing and both fat-burning and calm are blocked.

The calming, antianxiety sex hormone progesterone is typically low due to too much cortisol (stress hormone) and too much estrogen (from food, the environment, and liver recycling, which is often the result of the regular reliance on alcohol to 'relax' in the evenings after being so amped up during the day – more on this in a moment – and as a result, the mad rush feelings and the overreaction to things tends to be worse in the lead-up to menstruation. Throw in some sugary snacks and perhaps more caffeine when the afternoon exhaustion kicks in, and you have a cocktail of behaviors aimed at reducing stress that are in fact adding a significant level of stress to your body.

On top of the physical stressors are the emotional responses that do not serve us and keep us in an SNS-dominant state. As children, these emotional patterns probably protected us in some way but as adults they are often detrimental to our mental and therefore our physical health, and often our personal growth. I've listed a few of the most common emotional patterns I observe in rushing women below.

An inability to say no

I have heard the following words countless times from female clients and friends, 'I don't know how to say no.' There are many times in our lives when we want to say no but instead we say yes, usually to please other people and keep the peace. We want others to like us and we behave as if saying no sometimes will either lead them to believe we don't like them or make them think we are a terrible person. And when we spell it out on paper like this, you can see how crazy it is.

A client recently shared a great example of this pattern with me. She was scheduled to go into the hospital to have a baby and she had one day of solitude planned, the day before she was to give (cesarean) birth. Her older children were going to be at school and she simply wanted one peaceful day at home by herself to reflect and rest and be. So when her neighbor asked if my client could look after her sick child for a few hours while she went to a meeting, my client said yes... and begrudged her neighbor for asking. Yet if she had simply said no, or explained her plans for the day, it would have given her neighbor an opportunity to explore other options. Our no gives others the opportunity to grow.

It is time to stop giving up what you want in order to keep the peace. Sure it is lovely to give. Contributing to the world and those around you is a fundamental need for humans... contribution helps give our lives meaning and it fosters a harmonious community. Yet when we do it at our own expense and say yes when secretly we wish we'd said no, it doesn't serve anybody.

This pattern, the inability to say no, is a major drain on our energy, not to mention our time. It revs up our stress response, driving us in to, or holding us in SNS dominance. And our adrenal glands, which release the stress hormones, can also be significantly impacted upon over time. It is crucial to learn to say no. However, knowing that this will help your health is usually not enough to promote change. You will tell yourself you need to say no far more often than you currently do, yet your subconscious drive to avoid pain (the perceived loss of love from those asking things of you) will usually lead you back to being a yes girl.

Reflect

We'll delve deeper into the psychology of why we say yes in a later chapter but for now grab a pen and paper, and note down the things you regularly say 'yes' to, when you'd rather say 'no.'

Seeking acceptance, approval, appreciation, and love

Another way the above words could be phrased is 'seeking to avoid rejection' or 'to avoid being ostracized.' When we constantly aim to prove our worth to the people in our lives or those we meet, it is exhausting and adds another layer of stress to our busy lives. However, what I've noticed in my practice is that at first the woman can't reconcile her behavior with wanting to fit in, be accepted, and thought of as a good person. And then the penny drops... you can see it in her face, and the best way I can describe the expression is relief. And she looks lighter, freer somehow.

To come into awareness, you often have to look down upon a situation, as if you were an angel watching from above with an attitude of curiosity rather than any form of judgment or preconceived ideas about what might be going on. Then you see the situation as it really is, and that you simply said or did what you did to be accepted, approved of, appreciated, and ultimately loved. And there is nothing wrong with wanting any of those things. But when you are aware of what drives you, you also see that the behavior harms you in some way – for example, stresses you out and keeps you in SNS dominance – then you know you have the power to change it. When we don't know why we do what we do, then we can always seem to end up doing things we don't want to do, or perhaps feeling unappreciated, unhappy, and exhausted.

Reflect

You are lost without a map. Look down upon your precious self as a neutral observer and note down what you see as the path out.

Not putting you first

On an airplane the safety video instructs you put on your own oxygen mask first before helping others, because if you pass out due to lack of oxygen you will not be able to assist others. It is very easy to pay lip service to this concept and another matter entirely actually to act on it. When you go to meditate or practice yoga or go to a café to read your favorite magazine, you are taking care of you and nurturing your soul, and this helps everyone around you.

Typically, we are able to behave in a much calmer and kinder manner when we create a sense of spaciousness in our lives. When people tell me they have no time, of course I know they are busy. What I also know is that they have no space in their mind to fit in another task, another thing to remember. It is headspace women need, and only you can give yourself that. We make time for what we prioritize. Take the example of my girlfriend who started dreading picking her five children up from school.

> Every day was chaos and the boys are at that age where they smell after school and it was just so loud for the 20-minute drive home that I'd feel so stressed by the time we got there, I'd end up screaming at them on a daily basis. I couldn't cope and yet I felt like such a dreadful mother for yelling at them. One day, to prepare myself for the school pickup, I listened to spa music while I drove and it was on when the older children got into the car. After initially teasing me about my taste in music and making a few 'Om' noises, we had the calmest drive home we'd had since they hit puberty. So now that's part of my daily ritual. It doesn't always completely negate the chaos but it's certainly much less and I, too, am different. I'm not drowning now. I respond to them differently, from a much more centered space.

• • • • • • • • • • • • • • • • • •

Reflect

How could you incorporate relaxation rituals into your everyday life? Don't wait until you actually feel stressed.

Guilt

Guilt is such a futile emotion. Most often it is due to the perception that you have let someone else down. Yet when you pause to think about that, it is simply a story you are telling yourself. The reality is that it is not physically possible to let another human being down. If you do or say something, it is the other person's choice entirely whether they feel disappointment or any other emotion. And their response is 100 percent based on their conditioning, their life experiences up until now, just as yours is. You have never walked in anyone else's shoes, nor have they walked in yours. You have no idea what it is like to be them or what emotional patterns they run. If they choose disappointment, it is their choice. It is just an emotion and it will pass.

Many women feel guilty because they believe they are not a good enough friend, partner, wife, mother, daughter, sister, colleague... but it gets us nowhere. The first step to changing your exhausting emotional responses, the ones that don't serve you, is awareness. And although you may still feel guilt, you can catch yourself. You can recognize much sooner that you've responded to a situation with guilt and rather than letting it linger and permeate your life, your relationships, and your self-esteem, you can realize you have simply told yourself your old story. Make this one of your mental go-to statements... only if I indulge in the debilitating, exhausting, health-depleting emotion of guilt will I feel it, instead of remembering that I haven't walked in anyone else's shoes, cannot control how they will respond to my words or actions, and that only I determine how I feel.

Reflect

What leads you to feel guilty? From this point on, begin to become aware of the stories you tell yourself. They are simply that.

How women become SNS dominant

There are numerous roads to an SNS-dominant life, and some of them involve a high or low level of a particular physical substance, such as caffeine or progesterone, while others are the result of our emotional landscape and behaviors, which are 100 percent due to our beliefs. The trouble is, most of us are totally unconscious about what we really believe. Later chapters will offer assistance with the emotional side of things, but in the meantime here follows a summary of the physical aspects of lifestyles that can lead to SNS dominance.

Caffeine

I wish it weren't so, believe me! Caffeine is the fastest and surest way to amp up that SNS response. And how many people start their day with a caffeinated beverage? More than 90 percent of people in the West consume caffeine every day. It is a powerful nervous-system drug and also drives the adrenal glands to produce adrenalin (see page 16). Like stress, caffeine demands your body use glucose as its fuel, drawing on glucose in the blood or drawing the stored version of glucose (glycogen) out of the liver and the muscles into the blood to be used as the fuel in this highly alert state. The body doesn't like high circulating levels of glucose in the blood as it can damage the vessel walls. If the adrenalin had been made to literally get you out of danger, you would utilize the glucose in your fight or your escape. But typically, we are sitting at a computer screen while consuming caffeine, and with very little glucose utilization. In that state, your body must make another hormone, called insulin, to move the glucose out of the blood. Insulin is another fat-storage hormone and this is one of the mechanisms that links stress as a risk factor for type 2 diabetes.

What I've observed in so many women is that if their day is calm, non-chaotic and without pressure or demands, and caffeine is thrown into that mix, then the caffeine still stimulates (as that is its mechanism of action), but not to the point of overwhelm... and overwhelm can show up as snappy, impatient behavior or sadness and withdrawal. But how do you know when a day may present with challenges and therefore if it might be 'safer' to have a caffeinated drink? One client described it beautifully.

I like to start my day with a latte that I make myself. I sometimes then buy a coffee mid-morning when I'm out and about. If I don't speak to anyone all day, I feel OK. I do notice my energy crashes about two hours after the second coffee, but as far as the feelings of overwhelm go, they don't kick in. But these days, at the age of 41, I only have to get a phone call from my husband, and if he is panicked about something or seems frustrated with me, I can't stop shaking on the inside after I hang up. I feel like the smallest task on my to-do list is overwhelming and I make mountains out of molehills for the rest of the day. I even end up in tears feeling like I can't cope when I felt fine when I woke up.

When I came to see you about my periods, you asked me to take a break from coffee for two menstrual cycles. Not only did my premenstrual tension (PMT) go away but those feelings – even when my husband was worked up – didn't arise the whole time I was off coffee. I can't tell you the difference it has made to my day and to my health. I now have one coffee on the weekend, if my husband and I take the children out for breakfast, but it took that break for me to realize that coffee was the straw that broke this camel's back!

• • • • • • • • • • • • • • • • • • •

Action

Take the load off your SNS by taking a break from coffee. At first, switch to green tea, which contains caffeine (about 30mg per cup) but much less than coffee (about 80mg in a single shot, espresso-based drink), plus it is rich in antioxidants, has significant anticancer properties, and benefits the liver. Some rushing women find that even green tea is too stimulating, so once you have weaned off coffee using green tea, you can switch to herbal teas that contain no caffeine. Dandelion tea is also a great coffee alternative. Or simply make warm water with a squeeze of fresh lemon juice as your hot drink.

Low progesterone

When a woman's sex hormones are out of balance, it can feel like the world will end. She can feel 'out of her body,' as if she has no grounding and like there's something wrong but she doesn't know what it is. Progesterone clearly has a reproductive role in the body; however, it plays many other roles as well.

Progesterone behaves like an antidepressant and an antianxiety agent, and it is crucial for clear thinking. In the 18 years I have worked with people one-on-one about their health and nutrition, I have seen six women with optimal progesterone levels – six in 18 years! I know I see a biased group of the population... no one comes to see a health professional like me when they feel fabulous and everything in their world is perfect.

However, it does seem to have become common, but not normal, for a woman's progesterone to be low and that can mean any or all of the following:

- Low mood

- Unexplained weight gain

- An inability to lose weight despite excellent food and movement patterns

- Challenges conceiving

- Fluid retention

- Poor thyroid function

Low progesterone can also cause unexplained feelings of anxiety. And then it is difficult to discern if the feelings of overwhelm or the anxious feeling came first or if something is causing that.

From a scientific perspective it could be either. It can be that all of the rushing brought on the anxious feeling, as year after year living your life as a rushing woman is a surefire way to deplete your progesterone levels. My point is, however, that low progesterone levels can also lead us to the rush as progesterone physically helps to keep women calm. It is a classic chicken or egg situation.

Action

Do you think low progesterone might be playing a role in how you feel? If so, use a pen and paper to capture the aspects of your lifestyle that might be leading to this. Is it your regular overconsumption of caffeine, your perception of pressure and urgency, or knowing that you are in the wrong relationship for you? Some of these things you might be able to alter easily while others may require deep reflection and contemplation and therefore more time to decide if/when changes need to be made.

Lack of sleep

There are a few things I link to amazing health. Optimal nutrition, of course, fresh air, movement, love, forgiveness, and great sleep. Sleep affects our physical and mental health. One link that is particularly relevant to many of us is that between good-quality sleep and stress management.

Sleep is often the only time our bodies are able to access the rest-and-repair part of our nervous system (the PNS). Sleep is critical for skin regeneration, immunity, hair growth, nail growth, and all other non-vital processes the body will not prioritize during the day, particularly when under constant stress and SNS activation. For many of us, when we put our head on the pillow at night, it may be the first time that day we feel we have truly stopped. Yet the more tasks that pile up on our to-do list, the more we tend to sacrifice the one thing that allows our PNS to become dominant again... sleep.

When I ran programs at health retreats, I would often ask people what they loved most about their week. One of the most common answers I received was 'sleep.' Going to bed at a good time and getting up at the same time each morning, usually with the sun, sends a powerful message to your endocrine system, the system that involves all of the glands that regulate your incredibly important bodily functions like reproduction and the stress response. When you don't sleep enough, you don't allow your PNS to have as much of a chance to be the dominant arm of the nervous system. So for people who live their lives with an urgency, a hurriedness that their friends and colleagues may or may not witness (many women hide the panic away inside), the time they are asleep may be the only time they give their PNS the opportunity to drive the ship.

Yet many SNS-dominant women can't sleep properly or they do not feel sleep restores them. Remember that when you are in an SNS-dominant state, your body tends to churn out stress hormones and if one of those stress hormones is screaming to every cell of your body that your life is in danger, which is what adrenalin does, your body will never let you sleep deeply because it wants you to survive the imminent attack it perceives. So it is a vicious cycle. Sleep is difficult to restore to excellent quality, if you don't first allow the PNS to become the dominant arm of the nervous system.

Action

Try to get to bed early – at least three nights a week before 10 p.m. If you find that you suffer from scratchy or disturbed sleeps then you might find that simple sleep hygiene can improve your sleep while you work on overcoming being SNS dominant. Avoid caffeine after midday. Don't look at technology or watch stimulating TV shows before bed, make sure your bedroom is well aired – leave a window open if this will help. Most importantly, leave your mobile phone and any other technology on the other side of the door.

Over-exercising

As mentioned earlier, certain types of exercise can seem like more stress to an already overstressed human body. Do you think our ancestors woke up and thought it would be a great day for a run? No! Running meant we were attempting to escape from danger back then, while now it has become a way to burn off the excesses a Western lifestyle 'affords' us. I'm not saying running is bad, for those of you who love it. Barefoot running, in particular, promotes being present in the moment, while interval sprinting better mimics historical movement patterns and doesn't drive SNS dominance. There is also a science that can be applied to running to promote fat-burning and nervous-system calm, via how you eat, think and train. I'm simply saying that if running and high-intensity exercise (combined with good eating) hasn't shifted your weight by now, it is not suddenly going to start doing so until some other work on your body's chemistry and nervous system is done.

Even though you know you are just exercising intensely, from your body's perspective, once the threat (perceived by your body to be present due to the release of stress hormones) is dealt with, the PNS slows our heart rate and respiration back down, brings the blood back to the digestive tract so that we can digest our food, works to repair any tissue damage, and increases libido. Nighttime is when the PNS has lots of time to do its job. As you know now, the sympathetic and parasympathetic systems are supposed to balance each other nicely, and in those people who have a balanced nervous system, high-intensity exercise will lead to fat loss, as the parasympathetic rest time between workouts is when muscle tissue is built.

Those who are unable to lose fat by doing regular high-intensity exercise may have a dominant SNS, and, consequently, an inhibited PNS. This is due to too much systemic stress in the body, and for those people adding high-intensity exercise is counterproductive, as it adds to their sympathetic load, pushing them even more out of balance.

Action

Decrease your sympathetic load by reducing stressors and choosing an exercise that is done slowly and with the breath, such as Stillness Through Movement, restorative yoga, qi gong, tai chi, yoga, or the Feldenkrais Method. These activities increase the parasympathetic system and help balance the ANS. The goal is to balance the nervous system so that when you do need to rush, you can, but then you can leave the rush, and all its health-depleting effects, behind.

Lack of solitude

Another factor that can lead to SNS dominance is a lack of solitude. When I talk about being alone I don't mean feeling lonely. In fact, science has demonstrated some of the health benefits that come from spending time in solitude include decreased stress hormones, improved memory, creativity, mood, and empathy. It allows us to recharge.

On the inside this means that the PNS gets to have its time in the sun being dominant, where the vital rest, repair, and digest processes can do their work. When we rest and repair the body is able to choose between sugar and fat as its fuel, and it usually chooses both. That is a good thing. Health problems can occur when the body feels as if it has no choice but to always choose glucose for its fuel.

Action

How can you seek solitude in your day? Going for a walk by yourself and noticing the nature around you is a great place to start. If you live with other people and you have the house to yourself, even if it is only once a week for a brief period of time, allow yourself to stop for at least some of that time, even though you will likely feel like 'making the most of it' to get more jobs done.

You may feel that I cannot possibly understand your life and how busy you are. But part of what I want to show you is that when you create spaciousness in your life, you feel like you have more time, and you no longer have to rush. It may not feel possible for you right now, and particularly if you have small children. Often when they rest you need to rest, too. Although so many women rush around even more while their baby sleeps, to get on top of the jobs that have piled up! One way to look at it is to give yourself permission to rest on two out of the seven days of the week, while your baby sleeps. For the other five, you can choose to do tasks or rest. Or you may prefer to start with one day of rest and increase this by an additional day every second week, until you have three rest days a week. Small steps can feel much more manageable.

Another important thing to consider is that children are little for such a relatively short time. If you feel like right now you just can't take some time in solitude, you will soon be able to. If you feel like this then perhaps while they sleep, you can at least sit for five minutes and focus on your breathing. More begets more remember? It can be practical to start small with your solitude if you feel like it is a far-off dream.

Excess liver loaders

In my book *Accidentally Overweight* one of the nine factors I link to using body fat for fuel is optimal liver function. Without going into great detail here, I simply want you to know that some foods and certain beverages can instigate a stress response. Many women tell me, for example, that once they go to bed after drinking alcohol, they can feel their heart racing. Start to notice what affects you. The main liver loaders are:

- Alcohol

- Caffeine

- Trans fats

- Sugars, including fructose and sucrose

- Synthetic substances, such as pesticides, medications, skin 'care'

- Infection, for example viruses such as glandular fever (Epstein-Barr virus, Mononucleosis)

Most of these substances you have a choice about ingesting, the infection is something you have less control over. You know when you are regularly consuming too much when it comes to alcohol, caffeine, and refined sugars in your diet – and I mean too much for you. Each of us has a unique level of tolerance for each substance and you will know better than anyone if you are overconsuming something.

If something has welled up inside you, as you're reading this, your body's wisdom is trying to communicate with you. Knowledge is one thing; taking action on that knowledge is something entirely different. A period of time where you take action to reduce or abstain from liver loaders can make a vast difference to the rush and its consequences on your health. Plus, optimal liver function leads to better sex hormone balance, as you will soon read.

Alcohol is a big issue for many rushing women. Many are exhausted, overwhelmed, and haven't had any time to themselves for at least five or 25 years. I ask women who drink every night to finish the following sentence, 'Alcohol is...' And here follows some of the things they say:

- 'My only pleasure in the day.'

- 'The only way I can relax at the end of the day.'

- 'Something for me... the only thing just for me in my day.'

- 'The only way I get any peace.'

- 'Reward for all of my efforts over the day.'

The reality is that alcohol is none of those things. These are meanings that we give to alcohol. These are the stories you tell yourself about why you need it, why it is OK to have it every night of your life. I don't believe the human body, for women in particular, was designed to consume alcohol most nights of its adult life. And women are experiencing the consequences of regular overconsumption, with this type of drinking now highly associated with five of our biggest cancers. The links are undeniable. But for many of you, even scientific fact that the regular overconsumption of alcohol (amounts outlined later) significantly increases your risk of breast cancer won't stop you from telling yourself that it is your 'only pleasure in the day.' But seriously, if the only thing you derive pleasure from in your entire day is an alcoholic drink, then perhaps it is time for a new perspective. As an aside, many women repeat the same statements to me about coffee or a particular type of food. This is not about taking away your fun or your pleasure but being able to choose how much and how often you consume these liver loaders, rather than your desire for them being ruled by your emotional state... for then you feel out of control and often regret your food or drink choices.

Choice

We have so much to be thankful for. I encourage you to be truly thankful every day for the privilege of living in a peaceful country. Every night before you go to sleep, take a moment to be grateful simply for what you do have and not worry about what you may not. Take some time out every day to have an 'attitude of gratitude.' We are so blessed to live in a society where we have an amazing array of choices available each day... more than our ancestors would ever have dreamed possible. And, it is likely that anyone reading this, no matter how they may perceive their own life at present, still has a lifestyle that millions in the world would wish could be theirs. Many people don't have fresh water to drink. It's also easy to take choice for granted particularly when life doesn't work out quite the way we had planned. We have opportunities to shape our future but we don't always have control over unexpected events. We would never consciously choose for ourselves or those we love to have an accident, a serious illness, job loss, or to be involved in a natural disaster. But, even if challenges present themselves, we must never forget that we retain control over our attitude toward that event. When I talk with people about their perception of choice, I am fascinated, occasionally saddened, but mostly inspired by the immense power of the human spirit. Here is one such response:

> When my parents died when I was 16, I had no choice in the circumstance. However, I was faced with other choices... to seek the so-called comfort of drugs or the true support of friends, to be negative or positive, to look backward or forward. Although I had absolutely no choice surrounding the situation I found myself in, I still had a choice in terms of what attitude I adopted. I knew that whatever choice I made wouldn't bring them back so I simply chose to get on with my own life as best I could. Admittedly, there were times when I doubted I would succeed in doing so but there is no comparison between that which is lost by not succeeding and that which is lost by not trying.

> With no family to fall back on, or blame, I learned earlier than most that I was totally responsible for my own choices for the rest of my life. Because of the volunteer work I've ended up doing in the later part of my life, I've walked the beat with police as rocks were hurled at us, been called to an armed robbery, intervened in domestic violence situations, and sat for hours on a drug bust. Perpetrators of those crimes made different choices than me but I suspend judgment because I may have made the same choices once, and I give thanks that I didn't. Choices have given me more than my fair share of joy and sorrow. But even in my darkest moments, I remind myself to give thanks for that freedom to choose.

● ● ● ● ● ● ● ● ● ● ● ● ● ● ● ● ● ● ●

Every day, I am truly grateful for so much in my life, such as fresh air, freedom, and real food. I'm equally grateful for the things I don't have, like persecution, hunger, and disease. Every day, it is worth reminding yourself that the choices are yours. I cannot encourage you enough to spend time each day focusing on the things for which you are grateful. Share that gratitude with others. And remember to include the things that aren't in your life for which you are grateful too. As Tony Robbins so accurately says, 'What you focus on is what you feel.' If you tell yourself that alcohol is the only pleasurable thing in your entire day, then it will be – yet there is so much more on offer, around you and within you every minute of every day and night. It is just that when you are exhausted and running on the caffeine, sugar, alcohol highway of sub-optimal nutrition and SNS dominance, racing around everywhere with your to-do list never being all checked off, it can be quite a challenge to remember how magnificent your life truly is.

When you allow the PNS to be dominant – whether that's by drinking less caffeine, sorting out your sex hormone balance, going to bed earlier, scheduling some 'yin' type movement in your day, or exploring and resolving elements of your emotional landscape – you begin to experience more wellbeing and spaciousness. In addition, when you are PNS dominant, you not only see the magnificence and the wonder, but you can also feel it within, just as you did as a very little girl. Your rituals create your life. Get some good ones!

Life a long time ago... and life today

There is an age-old inclination wired into us to protect, hoard, and defend. The enemy is lurking, waiting to eat you, annihilate you. The part of our brain linked to the fight-or-flight response, which I described earlier, is part of the reptilian brain – despite being augmented by the limbic brain (a different part of the brain linked to emotions) and the neocortex (yet another part of our very clever brain) – and it is still focused on physical survival. And when we allow our most basic impulses – the very ones that helped the earliest humans survive – to direct the higher brain center, we act like lizards. And given we were born with the inclination to do whatever is needed to survive, we need to respect the genius of a brain that has done its job and brought us this far. But we also need to update our wiring since the chances of being eaten by a lion are slim. Even though we just rush, our body's perception is that that big cat is actually very real!

Being on red alert has now become maladaptive because it causes us to live in a constant state of tension, which is unhealthy and therefore counterproductive to our survival. Only our nervous system, of which our brain is a part, hasn't been able to keep up with the rate of change or the pace of life the West now asks of us. So for now, until our evolution can catch up (can it ever?), we have to choose to support the part of our nervous system that dissolves tension as long as we make it feel like it is safe to do so.

There is a wonderful analogy I love to use to describe how people have become oblivious to the stress and pressure in their lives. The origin of the following anecdote is unknown but it is thought to be based on a scientific experiment published in 1897. It is about a frog and as green tree frogs just happen to be one of my favorite creatures on the planet (and one of my nicknames is Frog), it appeals to me even more!

If you put a frog in cool water it swims around very happily. If you put a frog in boiling water it immediately jumps out to save itself. But if you put a frog into cool water and slowly bring that water to the boil, the frog doesn't notice and doesn't jump out.

I believe that most people in the West would jump out of the pressure in their lives, if they were suddenly thrown into it. But we don't jump out when it gradually increases over the years. We don't tend to notice until calamity hits. Don't let a health crisis wake you up to the fact that without your health you have nothing. If you recognize that you are like a frog whose world has been on the boil, act now to change it. Begin to put strategies in place to change either your situation or your perception of your life, or both. Either way, the changes it will foster in your biochemistry, your emotional landscape, and hence your health, are potentially enormous.

Reflect

Take a moment and consider how different your life would be if you were able to greet each day with more energy, feeling calmer and more able to practice patience and kindness? How would that make you feel?

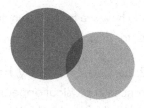

Chapter 3

Introducing Hormonal Havoc

The Impact of Rush on Your
Endocrine System

B efore we get to the aha moments that will help you understand
what might be going on in your body, you need a little bit of
science made simple to help you on your way... and it all starts with
the endocrine glands.

The endocrine system is made up of numerous glands that secrete
hormones, including:

- Pituitary

- Thyroid

- Parathyroids

- Adrenals

- Reproductive organs; the ovaries in women and the testes in
  men

Although the latter two are technically not endocrine glands
exclusively, for the purpose of explaining the role of the endocrine

system, their vital roles in how we feel and function on a daily basis, are important to understanding RWS.

Around the age of 12, as we enter puberty, boys and girls start to develop striking differences in physical appearance and behavior. Perhaps no other period in life so clearly demonstrates the impact of both the nervous system and the endocrine system in directing development and regulating body functions. Changes in the brain and pituitary gland markedly increase the synthesis of new messenger molecules, the sex hormones, from the gonads. In girls, fatty tissue starts to accumulate in the breasts and hips. At the same time, or a little later, in boys, protein synthesis increases, muscle mass builds, and the longer, larger vocal cords start producing a lower-pitched voice. These changes provide just a few examples of the powerful influence of the secretions from endocrine glands.

Coordination of the nervous and endocrine systems

Together, the nervous and endocrine systems coordinate functions of all body systems. The nervous system controls homeostasis (the point where all things are in balance) through nerve impulses, while the endocrine system releases its messenger molecules (called hormones) into the bloodstream.

The circulating blood then delivers hormones to virtually all the cells throughout the body. The nervous and endocrine systems are coordinated as an interlocking supersystem, referred to as the 'neuroendocrine system.' Certain parts of the nervous system stimulate or inhibit the release of hormones from the glands of the endocrine system. Hormones may then, in turn, promote or inhibit the generation of nerve impulses. Also, several molecules act as hormones in some locations and as neurotransmitters in others.

The nervous system causes muscles to contract and glands to secrete more or less of their products. The endocrine system alters metabolic activities, regulates growth and development, and guides reproductive processes. It therefore not only helps regulate the activity of things like smooth and cardiac muscle and some glands, it significantly affects virtually all other tissues in the body as well.

Nerve impulses tend to produce their effects within a few milliseconds. While some hormones can act within seconds, others can take up to several hours or more to bring about their responses. Also, the effects of stimulating the nervous system are generally brief compared with those of the endocrine system.

So with that out of the way, let's get into the details of how the endocrine system affects you; how you look, feel, and function every day, as well as the symptoms you may be experiencing, which signal that additional support in this area is needed and what benefits support will bring.

Firstly I want you to know that the pituitary gland, housed inside a part of your brain, is the master gland, or the switch of the endocrine system. Technically the hypothalamus – an organ with some endocrine tissue within it – influences the function of the pituitary; however, for ease of explanation and to keep the Rushing Woman's Syndrome message concise, the hypothalamus is only discussed briefly in Chapter 7 (see page 121).

The pituitary gland sends the signals out to your other endocrine system glands, alerting them to the hormones they need to make. Likewise, the thyroid talks to the ovaries. The adrenals and the ovaries also have a relationship and on and on the chatter inside you goes. That's what hormones do... they talk... they send messages, and each of those messages communicates information to the different cells, tissues, and organs inside your body. Nothing, and I mean nothing, works alone. Everything is influenced by something else.

So the importance of the coming sections – about the adrenal glands and the stress hormones they make, the ovaries and the sex hormones they make, the thyroid gland and the temperature-controlling, metabolism-influencing hormones it makes, as well as the master of them all, the pituitary – is enormous and will open your mind and your heart to a whole new way to view your health and the pace of our lives, as well as provide you with insights and support to make the changes you feel inspired to make. Hormonal systems parts I, II, III, and IV here we come!

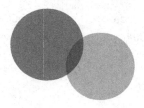

Chapter 4
Hormonal Havoc Part I: Down and Depleted
The Impact of Rush on Your Stress Hormones

There are different stages of stress: the alarm phase where adrenalin is high – covered in the previous chapter – is followed by an increase in cortisol, and the final stage when cortisol levels drop. When the body constantly cycles through the fight-flight-depletion cycle, this can, over time, result in weight gain (but not always), and affect our ability to feel calm and content, have good energy, be able to bounce out of bed every morning, and keep inflammation and stiffness away, as well as affecting our perceptions.

The symptoms are different depending on the stage of stress, but here follow some indicators that your body may need support in this area.

- You feel stressed regularly and like you are on red alert.

- You have gained weight during or after a stressful period; you may have lost weight initially during the stress but you regained that weight plus more.

- Your body fat has increased around your middle, back of your arms and you have grown what I lovingly refer to as a 'back veranda.'

- You have sugar cravings.

- You love coffee, energy drinks; anything that contains caffeine.

- You startle (jump) easily.

- You don't sleep well.

- You often wake up feeling unrefreshed or like you've been hit by a bus.

- You feel better if you can sleep until 8–9 a.m., rather than rising 5–7 a.m. (Many of you won't have been able to assess this as you don't have a choice about what time you get up).

- If you don't go to sleep by 10 p.m., you get a second wind and end up staying awake until at least 1 a.m.

- You regularly feel tired but wired.

- You retain fluid.

- Your face looks 'puffy' or swollen at times (and other causes have been ruled out).

- You are a worrier; you don't relax easily.

- Your family/friends tell you that you are a 'control freak.'

- Your body feels heavy and achy at times even though you don't have a medical condition that warrants this.

- You have high blood pressure.

- You have low, or the low end of normal, blood pressure.

- You get dizzy easily, but particularly when you go from sitting to standing quickly.

- You feel anxious easily.

- You tend to a low mood with no known other cause.

- Your breathing tends to be shallow and quite fast.

- You experience 'air hunger' (and other causes have been ruled out).

- You struggle to say 'no.'

- You laugh less than you used to.

- You feel like everything is urgent.

Your adrenal glands are two walnut-sized glands that sit just above your kidneys. Don't let their size trick you, they are powerful players in your overall health and, when functioning well, gift us with energy and vitality.

The adrenal glands are responsible for producing many hormones, two of which are your stress hormones – adrenalin, which I described in Chapter 2 (see page 16), and cortisol.

Cortisol – friend or worst nightmare?

Cortisol is your long-term stress hormone. For our ancestors, long-term stress always revolved around food being scarce and came along with wars, famines or floods. Under these kinds of circumstances we didn't know when we might get our next meal. In the West today, our long-term stress has little to do with famine, war or floods. Instead, it tends to be linked with ongoing financial pressure, relationship or family concerns, and worries about our health and our weight.

When we consistently, day after day, worry and feel anxious about different aspects of our lives, it can easily become a chronic stress-hormone response that increases cortisol output. In turn this can slow down your metabolism and essentially change your behavior because your body is getting the message that it has to do everything at a rapid pace and you don't feel as though you can keep up.

Cortisol can either be your friend or your worst enemy so it's important to understand how it works. When made in optimum amounts, cortisol adds many wonderful health benefits. As one of the body's primary anti-inflammatory mediators, and having been converted into cortisone, it dampens down the effect of wherever inflammation is present in your body and stops your body from feeling rigid, stiff or in pain. That feeling that many people describe after coming out of difficult times of having suddenly aged is often the result of suboptimal cortisol levels during such periods. When present in the right amount, cortisol also buffers the effect of insulin, meaning that optimal amounts help you to access body fat as a fuel for energy while also inhibiting rapidly fluctuating blood sugar levels and maintaining better stability.

Your cortisol levels vary over the day. In the right amount, it assists you with various bodily functions throughout the course of the day. Optimally, cortisol levels will be high in the morning and it is one of the mechanisms that wakes you up and helps you bounce out of bed full of energy and vitality. Let's say, for the purpose of this discussion, that 25 units at around 6 a.m. are ideal. By midday, optimum cortisol will sit at around 15 units, and, by 6 p.m., levels will ideally be at around four units. By 10 p.m., optimum cortisol levels are around two units, and they stay at this level until around 2 a.m. when they begin to rise again, very slowly and steadily.

What your mother told you about how one hour of sleep before midnight is worth two after is absolutely true because as cortisol starts to rise after 2 a.m. the processes of rest and repair begin to slow down. The following graph illustrates this.

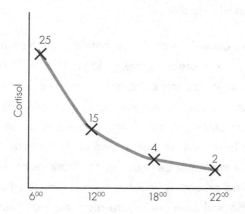

Figure 2: Optimal cortisol profile
Cortisol level is high in the morning and falls away again by the evening.

If you are in a state of chronic stress it begins to change the stress hormone profile of your body. In the early stages of long-term stress, evening cortisol levels start to spike again rather than continue to decline. At this stage, your morning cortisol levels are still optimal and you are able to bounce out of bed and get on with your day with a reasonable amount of energy. But with evening levels creeping up, good sleeping patterns can be interrupted.

With elevated cortisol levels, other changes in body chemistry begin to unfold. It has been suggested that elevated cortisol is the one common thread behind what has come to be described as metabolic syndrome; that is elevated blood pressure, elevated cholesterol, and insulin resistance. The latter condition (insulin resistance) acts as a warning sign that if nothing changes in the near future, type 2 diabetes is a likely consequence. If we remember that our bodies are entirely geared for survival and that cortisol tells every cell of your body that food is scarce, another of its roles is to slow down your metabolic rate. This slowed metabolism means that you burn body fat for energy far more slowly than you have in the past, as cortisol is designed to make sure that you survive this perceived period of famine.

We also spoke about how cortisol is 'catabolic,' which in technical terms means that it breaks protein down into building blocks, known as amino acids. This catabolism is one of the mechanisms through which cortisol slows your metabolism. As your muscles are made from proteins, cortisol signals them to break down, to provide your body with the fuel it perceives it needs to survive. Even though it might just be reacting to financial or relationship concerns milling around in your head while you're sitting in front of the TV, additional amino acids are also needed in the blood to help repair tissues. As a consequence of the catabolic signaling of cortisol, the amino acids can be converted, through a process called 'gluconeogenesis,' back into glucose (sugar), which your body does because it thinks it may be useful to assist you with your stress. The problem is, if you are not active, you won't utilize this increase in blood glucose and your body will need to secrete insulin to return your blood glucose levels to an optimum level and return the glucose in the blood to storage. Remember that glucose is stored as glycogen in the muscles and the liver.

But over time, the catabolic signaling of cortisol itself has likely broken some of your muscles down, so now there is less space for glucose storage. As a result, whatever can be returned to the remaining muscles is returned and the remaining glucose is converted into body fat. It is more important to your body to keep the glucose level of your blood in a normal range than to be concerned about whether you have wobbly bits around your middle! Essentially, in addition to a decreased ability to utilize fat as an energy source, too much cortisol dysregulates your blood sugar metabolism, which also makes you fat. This is one way in which cellulite can appear, since fat can now be deposited where muscles once were. It is also the process through which long-term stress can lead to type 2 diabetes.

Your body doesn't realize that the stress you are experiencing is not due to a lack of food in the world, it interprets the additional cortisol production as food scarcity and holds on to extra body fat because it instinctively knows that it has a greater chance of survival if it has more fuel stored. If you think about how people now understand the importance of not carrying too much body fat, whether for health reasons or vanity (or both), and may believe that eating less is the only solution to body-fat loss, you can begin to understand how cortisol can provide a potential challenge that gets in the way of our attempts at shedding body fat. Feeling like she is fighting an uphill battle with her body can be an immense source of stress for a woman, adding another layer of stress to her already hectic mind.

Understanding the cortisol problem

It doesn't matter how amazingly you eat or how much exercise you do, if cortisol is telling every cell of your body that food is scarce, and your metabolism slows down as a result, your clothes will slowly get tighter. Since cortisol is telling every cell in your body to store fat, it is very difficult, if not impossible, to decrease body fat until the cortisol issue is resolved. In order to begin utilizing body fat as a fuel, we must get to the heart of the stress and either change the situation or alter our perception.

Cortisol has a very distinct fat deposition pattern – you typically lay it on around your tummy. Once again, it is your body's quest for survival that governs this. If you think about it, if food suddenly did run out, your major organs have very easy access to fat (or energy) to keep you alive. You also tend to lay fat down on the back of the arms, and you grow what I lovingly call a back veranda.

To reiterate this important point: most people tend to go on a diet when they notice that their clothes are getting tighter. This diet generally leads you to eat less and therefore you reaffirm to your body that food is scarce and exacerbate your cortisol problem. But food is nowhere near scarce. In fact, it is abundant for you. If you decided at 3 a.m. that you wanted a pack of chocolate cookies, you could get them. So what you're really doing by eating less on your diet is confirming to your body what it perceives to be true and this only slows your metabolism even further.

Elevated cortisol coursing through your body presents another challenge for you as well. Since your body perceives that food is hard to come by, it's going to tell you to eat anything you can get your hands on and it becomes very difficult not to overeat. Regardless of how strongly you tell yourself just to stick to three corn chips when you get home from work, if that pack of crackers is open in front of you, cortisol will scream at you how lucky you are that there is food in front of you and to eat it all up before it disappears, and somehow before you know it, the whole pack is empty! Please don't get me wrong... of course willpower and self-discipline do have a place here. It is simply my intention to show you how the very ancient hormonal mechanisms operate and take over because they believe they know better than you when it comes to survival. If you learn how to decipher the messages it is communicating to you, your body can be an incredible teacher. And additional body fat is sometimes simply a vehicle of communication – just as an unjustified panicked perception of life is asking you to explore your biochemistry and your beliefs that allow this to be the case.

Silent stress

Not all of us are drama queens who are running around flailing their arms screaming, 'I'm so stressed, I'm so stressed!' Some of us are incredibly private and keep things under such a tight wrap that sometimes we don't even recognize ourselves that we've been in a stressed state for a long time. We're so busy presenting a happy face to the world that we're like the boiling frog that starts in cool water that gradually gets warmer and warmer (see Chapter 3, page 39). For some, the stress is silent.

When we feel privileged and grateful for all that we have in our lives, sometimes we find it difficult to complain about anything. A common internal phrase will be, 'There are so many people worse off than me.' When you think a thought along these lines, it immediately sets you up to feel guilty about what concerns you and you stop focusing on your source of stress. But by covering up the stress with a feeling of guilt, you don't ever get the opportunity to explore what is bothering you, and more importantly, why. So, although there are people worse off than you in this world, your thought is (of course) valid and you're missing an opportunity to transform your stress. We will explore the 'whys' at the heart of your stress in greater detail in Chapter 9 (see page 157). For now, I'll share a common example of keeping the peace. This will help you see how the perceptions we bring to our everyday lives can lead to cortisol from an emotional source being a contributor to your health challenges or your internal panic.

We know through basic psychology that humans will do more to avoid pain than they will ever do to experience pleasure. One common situation that showcases this perfectly is those people who will do anything to keep the peace and avoid conflict. When you're always walking around on eggshells around others, inwardly you become highly strung because you couldn't possibly let your guard down or relax. If, for example, this extends to your intimate partner who has a tendency to explode in angry outbursts that to you seem unpredictable, well hello silent stress hormone production! I have seen countless women who live like this.

For some women, avoiding feeling emotional pain comes in the form of eating too much or making other poor choices, such as drinking bucket-loads of wine or chain-smoking cigarettes. As alternatives, some people may cope with, or explore their pain by keeping a journal, going for a walk, a run, or a swim. Others might pray, meditate, or phone a friend and chat to deal with emotional pain. Some will do a combination of those that support our health and those that may potentially harm our health. And all of these activities may take place with or without a conscious understanding of why.

I want to help you see why, so you can change your response if it is hurting your health, especially if the stress hormone production triggered by your subconscious emotional responses is blocking either weight management or calm or both.

Worrying is no good for your health

Every day of my working life I work with people who eat too much. They are aware that they do and still they can't seem to stop. Sometimes that food is nutritious and sometimes it's not. Regardless, they know that their body and their health would be much better off if they stopped consuming food in the quantities they do.

Regularly, these women are coming to see me because they want to lose weight. They know what to eat and what not to eat to lose weight, yet they don't do it, even though they truly believe that they are desperate to lose weight. They are precious, intelligent people who don't understand why they do what they do.

You tell yourself that you would do anything to lose weight, to be slimmer. You probably have all the information you need to do this. So what's holding you back? Or what gets in the way once you've started?

There is a really big difference between a few mouthfuls of ice cream and the entire pint, between eating one cookie with your cup of tea in the evening and polishing off the whole pack. Eating too much not only makes our belly feel uncomfortable and overly full, it often leads us to say incredibly unkind things to ourselves like, 'I have no willpower, I can't believe how useless I am!' We know we shouldn't do what we do but we do it anyway, and it often leads us to go to bed feeling upset with ourselves; guilt-riddled to the point that we believe we'll never be able to change. A belief that things are permanent is very destructive.

So what might drive someone with the best of intentions to keep eating even though they know they shouldn't?

In addition to the elevated cortisol caused by long-term stress, there may be other biochemical factors involved. Things such as low progesterone (see Chapter 2, page 28), poor thyroid function, or blood sugar that surges and plummets all play a part and there are also likely to be emotional factors and core beliefs they probably aren't even conscious of.

The crux of it is, leave the worrying until something actually becomes a problem. Then, once it becomes a problem, you can face it, but worrying over something that may never eventuate only serves to harm you. The ripple effect of worries, through the production of excess cortisol, can very slowly and subtly change your metabolism to one of fat storage, consequently leaving your headspace full of sadness and withdrawn temperament. For some of you worry is at the heart of your rush. And it's the chemical signals created by your body, that your body believes will help you based on the information it is receiving, that are driving this.

Adrenal fatigue

If stress has been prolonged, the next biochemical stage of stress involves your cortisol falling low. Keeping in mind that your adrenal glands were not designed to sustain this kind of drawn-out stress, if you've had high cortisol levels for many, many years, your adrenal glands may not be able to keep up with the production levels your body is demanding and so they crash. In general terms, you burn out. The most common symptoms of this include:

- Difficulty getting up in the morning

- Inability to handle stress

- Regular and unexplained fatigue

- Cravings for salty foods

- Mild depression

- Insomnia

- A weak immune system, prone to recurrent infections

- Exhaustion in the mornings – but if you feel better at any stage of the day it is in the evenings. If you don't go to bed by 10 p.m. though, you'll likely still be awake at 1 a.m., as you get a second wind

- See also Chapter 2, page 15, as the result of RWS is often adrenal fatigue.

More recently, this has become known as adrenal fatigue, because the major symptom is a deep and unrelenting fatigue. Yet even though fatigue is the major symptom, I have observed in many women who experience this condition that though they are beyond tired, they are also wired. In this state of being tired but wired what you crave the most is a deep restorative sleep and yet quite regularly this eludes you.

Your adrenal hormone production is usually at the heart of this. But the pituitary gland, part of the endocrine system – and also responsible for the thyroid, parathyroids, and reproductive organs – is the mother gland (the hypothalamus is the master switch). So although treatment for adrenal fatigue usually involves a range of strategies that support the adrenals themselves, going one step further and assisting the pituitary (and also the whole of the endocrine system) can be immensely powerful and highly beneficial to restoring your health and vitality.

As you now know, the adrenal hormone cortisol is ideally high in the morning and the right amounts help you bounce out of bed. It plays a role in how vital you feel and helps the body combat any inflammatory processes that want to kick in. Stiffness is a key symptom of adrenal fatigue. For those with chronic stress, morning cortisol levels tend to be low, and, if 25 units is the ideal, with adrenal stress you may only get to 10 units. It can make it very difficult to get out of bed when you have such low levels and by mid-afternoon you'll likely be at an all-time low and feel as though you need to eat something sweet or consume something with caffeine to get through the afternoon (this can also be the result of low blood sugar or poor thyroid function, explored in a later section). For an adrenally fatigued person, cortisol is nice and low in the evenings (as it should be), but if you don't get to bed before 10 p.m., you will often get a second wind, and find it much harder to fall asleep, partly due to the body's natural adrenalin surge that tends to happen between 10:30 p.m. and 11:30 p.m. The following graph illustrates this cortisol pattern.

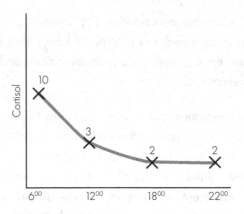

Figure 3: Typical cortisol profile in adrenal fatigue
Both the waking and midday cortisol readings are low.

It is likely that prior to the drop in cortisol, this adrenal hormone was high (although this is not always the case). However, just because your cortisol is low now doesn't mean you'll suddenly start burning fat for energy and find it easy to lose any surplus body fat, as this is due to cortisol's relationship with insulin, described previously (see page 50).

Since you're so exhausted you can barely get through your day, exercise may feel like the last thing in the world you want to do. If you push through this feeling and engage in cardiovascular exercise, you actually feel worse instead of getting the normal energy boost that exercise typically gives us. You get increasingly frustrated because you believe that eating less and doing cardio-based exercise is the only path to losing weight, and still you can't bring yourself to do either, despite the best of intentions. Every time you eat something sweet, you eat too much, or another month goes past without much movement. The transition in your head as you reflect on this may take you down a rabbit hole of guilt, saying mean things to yourself and silently giving up. You think 'who cares?' whenever you feel like eating something that won't really nourish you, and the not-so-great eating continues, especially an excess consumption of carbohydrates as you desperately search for energy. Your clothes keep getting tighter and this just adds to your stress. The vicious cycle is self-perpetuating.

As I've already mentioned, humans were never designed to sustain long-term stress, and our individual bodies cope with it in different ways. Some people will remain in an adrenalin-dominant stress-hormone scenario their entire lives, others will flip into a more cortisol-dominant stress response. If the stress response doesn't truly switch off, there is the potential that the adrenals will eventually crash, and cortisol output is no longer optimum or elevated. It will be negligible. At its extreme, this is a condition called Addison's Disease, yet if a person's cortisol level is extremely low but still falls just inside the 'normal range,' that person will be told that they are fine. They feel lousy but all the tests they have always come back 'normal.' They feel anything but normal, and people who know and love them will often comment that they are a shell of their former selves.

Cortisol can also be rather sinister in that it can interfere with your steroid (sex) hormone metabolism, your sleep patterns via its interference with melatonin, and also your mood via serotonin.

The serotonin–melatonin seesaw

Does this sound like your typical day? Healthy breakfast, mid-morning coffee, salad or sandwich for lunch... with probably something sweet to follow lunch, but other than that, you are quite proud of yourself when you reflect on your food consumption so far for the day.

If this sounds like you, I predict that many of you then fall into one of three categories later in the day. Do you:

1. Hit mid-afternoon and eat anything and everything in sight, and then spend the rest of the day kicking yourself because you started off so well?

2. Get so busy during the afternoon that food does not enter your head until you arrive home and a glass of white wine and possibly some cheese and crackers allows you to let out a sigh of relief that the day is winding down?

3. Or neither of the above and the free-for-all starts after dinner, when you find yourself standing in front of the fridge or pantry saying to yourself, 'I want something. I don't know what it is that I want but I want something. And maybe it's in here!'?

Perhaps all three apply to you!

Never fear, a new understanding is near.

The first two options are primarily about blood glucose. The third option describes serotonin – our happy, calm, content hormone. It makes us feel content with our lot in life, that there is nothing more that we could want in this world, and helps to keep panic at bay. Melatonin is our sleep hormone and is responsible for sending us to, and keeping us, asleep. Serotonin and melatonin work antagonistically; in other words when one goes up, the other goes down.

The mechanisms that govern a multitude of hormonal processes in our body are called circadian rhythms. These rhythms, alongside fading sunlight, allow melatonin to rise, and in turn, serotonin must fall.

When a hormone that makes you feel happy, calm, and content (serotonin) decreases, it can create a noticeable sinking feeling or an irritation – a distinct change in mood even though nothing in the external world has changed. Five minutes earlier you felt fine, yet now there is this nagging feeling that you want something; that something is amiss and you're not sure exactly what it is. This change in serotonin, which occurs as day becomes night, may be part of the reason many couples find themselves having 'big ticket item' conversations later in the day.

Our chemistry makes us feel like we want something and our brain tries to label what that might be. We usually don't find ourselves waking up and announcing that we absolutely must renovate the kitchen immediately! We keep those proclamations for evening and if you live with your significant other, they are more likely to be on the receiving end of a 'more intense tone' describing what you have decided is missing from your life at this time of day. Of course that can be a good thing!

Hormones are more powerful than you might realize and sometimes lie at the heart of the change in our headspace and mood, and also our food choices. Humans instinctively know that carbohydrate-rich foods promote serotonin production, which is partly why when the 'I want something' syndrome hits, many women head for the pantry. You hope what you want is in there. Often, though, guilt is all you find.

For someone in this pattern, mornings can also prove a challenge. Melatonin is destroyed by sunlight, which is one of the reasons why you tend to feel great all day when you go outside and exercise in the morning. The melatonin plummets when the retina of your eyes is exposed to light and, as a result, your serotonin surges. With a melatonin–serotonin seesaw hormonal profile, on a day where you get up and expose your eyes to sunlight, you can cope with almost anything. The flip side, though, is not so appealing. If you haven't gotten to bed before midnight, have slept poorly, or both, you may prefer not to rise with the sun, or small children, as you're not feeling well rested. If you don't actively seek sunlight and just wander out of bed sometime during the morning, your melatonin slowly seeps away, and your serotonin slowly rises. On a day like this it's likely you feel as though you need a hefty dose of caffeine to get you going.

Reflect

If you're nodding along as you read this because it sounds so familiar and the your evening 'carbfest' is out of control, the solution may not initially – or always – be purely dietary, so keep reading.

The first step is to start getting up at the same time every morning and going outside to engage in some form of movement. Welcome the day with tai chi, a walk, some stretches, preferably something breath-focused. If that is not possible because of your family situation, open the drapes and let the morning sun bathe you. Commit to doing this for four weeks, every day, and bring awareness to whether your evening carbohydrate cravings settle. Also notice if this helps any anxious feelings you may experience or that may intensify in the evenings. Your serotonin will love you for it.

Perceptions

As you can see, cortisol plays many roles in our body. Optimal levels are vital for burning body fat as fuel, feeling calm and content, good energy, being able to bounce out of bed every morning, and keeping inflammation and stiffness away. However, our perceptions also play a huge role in the stress response of our body, as past traumas or low-grade stress both take their toll on our wellbeing. I hope that the following messages will help you to open up to a new perspective on health, food, movement, life, feelings, your beliefs, and, so importantly, how calm and safe you feel in this world.

The importance of rest

You'll see from the solutions I offer in Chapter 11 that offering strategies to support you adrenally is at the heart of everything I do; and the desire for you to rest and to rest well, in a restorative and revitalizing way. Rest must follow action for us to have optimal health, excellent fat-burning, and the ability to remain calm, and very few of us these days truly rest, although we might believe we do. As outlined in the previous chapter, the PNS is active when we truly rest. This is the 'rest and repair' arm of our nervous system, but it can be dominated by the opposite arm of the nervous system, the sympathetic nervous system (see Chapter 2, page 18). The PNS also allows us to digest our food well and its activation is essential not only to feeling centered and calm, but to a tummy that isn't bloated after eating. Food is not supposed to bloat us yet a bloated stomach is a major complaint of more than 70 percent of women in the West. Calm is vital to optimal digestion, a topic covered later in Chapter 8. The following excerpts are from an article I wrote for a magazine about the role of stress in illness, which begins to explain some of the background to digestive system problems such as irritable bowel syndrome (IBS) and other health challenges.

Every moment, our brain is assessing the world around us and asking the question: 'Am I safe?' This question is asked on all three levels: intellectually, emotionally, and from a survival perspective. If at any moment the brain determines you are in danger on any of these three levels, it sends out an alert to the body and the fight-or-flight stress response occurs. Mechanisms of survival are activated by the brain stem to prepare you to face the situation or run away. This occurs whether we are being chased by a tiger, sitting for an exam, seeing flashing lights in our rearview mirror, or being spoken to in an inappropriate way. It occurs any time the brain perceives 'danger!'

All of these responses are appropriate to survive an attack from a tiger or any other danger. However, once the danger is gone and the stress is over, these body functions are designed to return to a state of balance. BUT! If during these stressful events the emotional brain or limbic system is involved (we feel fear, anger, resentment), it then sends a message to the brain stem to maintain the stress response to keep us safe, just in case such a situation ever happens again. Over time, this can develop into a chronic stress response even though we may not be able to recognize what led us to be stressed, given that often it is not an authentic threat to our life.

It is well recognized that 'stress' plays a major role in the development of many illnesses as does the food we feed ourselves. Consider the list of stress physiology responses and it is immediately apparent that long-term, these are the Western world's most common chronic ailments.

The following list outlines some common ailments and their biochemical relationship to stress. They include:

~ Adrenalin is released: anxiety

~ Blood glucose increases: type 2 diabetes

~ Blood pressure rises: hypertension

~ Pulse increases: cardiac arrhythmia

~ Muscles tense: neck and back pain

~ Pupils dilate: far-sightedness

~ Immunity downregulates: any immune-related diseases

~ Digestion is downregulated: irritable bowel syndrome, constipation, indigestion

~ Libido is downregulated: impotency, infertility

• • • • • • • • • • • • • • • • • •

The importance of diaphragmatic breathing

Science tells us that the only way we can consciously affect our ANS is with our breath, which is why it is the cornerstone of all my adrenal support solutions. If there is nothing else you take from this book, I want to encourage you with every cell in my body to get a ritual in your day that focuses on breathing well. This is the key to shifting many aspects of your chemistry including those driving you to switch from fat storage to fat burning and is crucial for cultivating calm.

Your breath lies at the heart of such powerful shifts in your nervous system and your biochemistry because the overarching role of the ANS is to perceive the internal environment. And, after processing the information in the central nervous system, it regulates its function. As the name 'autonomic' implies, it is independent of the conscious mind. Think about a family of ducks and their newborn ducklings. Just like those darling ducklings, the autonomic nervous system will always follow the leader, and the breath is the only part of the autonomic nervous system that can be controlled consciously. Your body follows your breath's lead. Breathing dominates your autonomic nervous system, and because you breathe 5,000–30,000 times a day – or two to five hundred million times in your lifetime – it has the potential to influence you positively or negatively in many ways.

There is nothing in this world that communicates safety more effectively to your body than your breath. Breathing in a shallow way, with short, sharp inhalations and exhalations, the kind of breathing we often engage in when we feel stressed, communicates to your body that your life is in danger. You have just learned about the cascade of hormonal events that follow such alarm and the role these hormones play in switching fat-burning on or off. Regardless of what led you to breathe shallowly in the first place – whether it was a deadline, your perception of pressure or a lifetime habit of your nervous system – how you breathe is also a fast track to the symptoms of anxiety and, potentially, panic attacks.

Long, slow breathing that moves your diaphragm, communicates that you are very safe. Nothing downregulates the production of fat-storage stress hormones or the alarm signals within your body more powerfully.

Practice diaphragmatic breathing by making sure your tummy moves in and out as you breathe, as opposed to just your upper chest. You can begin your breath by allowing the lower part of your tummy to expand and then imagine, as the breath slowly continues, that the expansion of your tummy has now extended into the area where you can feel your rib cage meet. You might like to place your hand on your tummy or across your diaphragm (just below your sternum) to anchor your breath down deep. Keep the slow inhalation going until your upper chest feels like it is pushing your ribs out at the sides of your body. Then, rather than hold your breath, pause and slowly allow the exhalation to begin in the reverse order of the inhalation with the top and side of the chest emptying first, followed by the middle of your abdomen and lastly your tummy. You may at first feel as though you're not able to get parts of your body to engage with this so please be kind and patient with yourself as this takes practice! The parts of you that have become disconnected will be thrilled to be back in touch.

Action

Schedule regular breathing intervals into your day until it becomes your new way of breathing (unless you do find yourself in a moment of danger that requires you to escape such as slamming your foot on the brake, if someone suddenly drives out in front of you!). Make appointments with yourself to breathe. Perhaps as you boil the kettle each morning (for your lemon hot water of course!), instead of racing around doing 50 tasks, stand in the kitchen and breathe – if your mornings are peaceful.

Do it numerous times over the course of your day and link it to daily routines like taking a shower to anchor it. Book a meeting into your calendar each afternoon at 3 p.m. If you work at a computer, have a reminder pop up on the screen that it is time for your meeting with yourself to do 20 long, slow breaths.

So often we don't prioritize our wellbeing and yet we keep appointments with other people so make sure you keep the appointments you make with yourself. There are also a number of movement activities that facilitate a strong breath focus like tai chi, qi gong, yoga (restorative yoga in particular), and these can be wonderful activities to engage in regularly.

For me personally, qi gong is one of the ways I choose to begin my day. It is not always easy to fit it in to a day with hourly meetings or appointments, but it is my habit now and has been for years. I had a period of time where I let this ritual go, however, and I soon learned how crucial it is to set up my day with a restoration-focused session. Without it my clarity, sex hormone balance, and vitality are not the same. The breath is the foundation pillar of calm and, therefore, of optimal health. It is practices such as these that allow us to quiet the stories that fill our minds and act as a constant source of stress.

The importance of laughter

Often we forget about this simple and free tool. Laughter can help us to powerfully transform our world. If we see life as tough, full of hard work, pain and drudgery, it will be precisely that. We see the world through unconscious filters that create our perspective of the world, whether we have a negative or positive outlook. I am not denying that life can be tough at times or suggesting that we shouldn't be honest if we feel down, but when we always see the world this way, and believe that it will never be any different, then it is likely that this is how it will be for us.

A belief that everything is always going to be hard and painful sends a dangerous signal to every cell of your body. Do your absolute best to shift your thinking to see life as an adventure, a journey, and a gift, full of opportunity, and a process through which you can contribute. Some of the greatest, most moving stories I have ever heard involved someone turning a horrific hardship into their greatest opportunity. Keep this in mind. Keep in mind, too, that you can choose to laugh at the calamity around you.

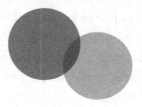

Chapter 5
Hormonal Havoc Part II: Menstrual Misery
The Impact of Rush on Your Ovaries and Sex Hormones

Another part of the endocrine system intimately involved in our capacity to feel calm, cope, and be happy involves the various glands and tissues that produce our sex hormones. In women, the ovaries are the main source of sex hormone production; however, both the adrenal glands and fat cells also make sex hormones. Other parts of the body do too, but in much smaller amounts. The body also contains tissues that produce hormones themselves but that are not sensitive to hormone levels in our body. The reason some tissues are hormone-sensitive and some are not relates to the presence of receptors for a particular hormone being present in that tissue. Let me explain.

Hormones and receptors: like locks and keys

For a hormone to elicit its effects, it has to bind to a receptor. This means that even though your body might make a certain hormone, it doesn't necessarily mean you get the great, or not so great effects, of that hormone. The easiest way to imagine how hormones interact with a receptor site is to picture a lock and key. When the key fits into the lock, you get the effects of the hormone. Breast tissue, for example, contains receptors for estrogen and progesterone, the two main female sex hormones, and is therefore highly sensitive to them.

In the correct balance, sex hormones are wonderful substances that give you energy and vitality. If you're not making enough sex hormones relative to your stage of life or if they are out of balance, they can also wreak havoc. Very few substances have the power to impact our body the way sex hormones do, especially when it comes to maintaining a sense of calm, mental clarity, the ability to be patient and not make mountains out of molehills, fat burning, beautiful skin, and fertility.

The main sex hormones we will cover in this chapter are estrogen and progesterone, with a particular focus on their role in body shape, size, fat burning, and inner peace, for when sex hormones are out of balance, this alone can have you feeling all pent-up with far too many places to go. First, here are some indicators that your body may need support in this area:

- You have heavy periods.

- Your menstrual flow contains clots.

- You have painful periods.

- You take painkillers during menstruation.

- You get a heavy, dragging feeling as the menstrual blood passes.

- You have swollen and/or tender breasts in the lead-up to menstruation.

- You experience mood swings in the lead-up to menstruation – or at the same time each month, for example around ovulation – which swing anywhere from immense irritability to intense sadness, sometimes in the same hour, and often for no reason you can fathom.

- You get PMS.

- You have regular headaches or migraines in the lead-up to menstruation.

- You have an irregular menstrual cycle.

- You are experiencing (or experienced) a debilitating menopause, such as sleeplessness and hot flushes (flashes) that are disruptive to your quality of life.

- You have PCOS, endometriosis or fibroids.

- You get skin breakouts before or during your cycle.

- You have acne, which started in puberty and hasn't resolved.

- You gained weight during puberty for the first time (can also be food-related and/or emotional).

- You have a tendency to a low mood – this occurred at puberty for the first time (can also be food-related and/or emotional).

- You experience fluid retention that worsens in the lead-up to menstruation.

- You experience anxiety in the lead-up to menstruation.

- You get food cravings, particularly for sugar, that increase in the lead-up to menstruation.

- You feel deep fatigue in the lead-up to menstruation.

- You are having challenges conceiving.

- You have unexplained infertility.

- Your bowel habits change (either to constipation or diarrhea) in the lead-up to or during menstruation.

- Your head feels 'foggy' in the lead-up to menstruation.

- Most months you have a day/s off due to menstruation challenges.

- You feel like you can't get your breath past your heart (and down into your belly) in the lead-up to menstruation.

- You have pimples/congested skin/acne on your back or chest.

- You have 'unexplained' weight gain, particularly around the abdomen and hips.

- You have cold hands and feet and this gets worse in the lead-up to menstruation.

- You have tendency to have yellow-tinged skin (that is not due to other factors, such as a liver disease).

- You experience poor (or worse) sleep quality in the lead-up to menstruation.

Can estrogen make you frantic?

Estrogen is a feminine hormone (that men also make in small amounts), and it has many important roles within your body. It is required for reproduction, supports cardiovascular health, and promotes new bone growth. When there is too much estrogen compared to other hormones, particularly progesterone, it can create myriad challenges. Estrogen can also be problematic if there is too much of one type of estrogen compared to other types.

From a female reproductive perspective, estrogen's main role is to lay down the lining of the uterus. It does this between days one to 14 of a typical 28-day cycle – day one is the first day of menstruation. The laying down of the lining during these first 14 days prepares the female body to conceive. Whether she wants it or not, estrogen wants a menstruating female to fall pregnant every single month of her life! Remembering that our bodies are completely geared for survival, the continuation of the human species is an integral part of that survival process.

This biological imperative to conceive each month prompts estrogen to ensure that there is adequate body fat to protect a fetus, as most females will not immediately know that they have fallen pregnant. If a woman is very slender and has insufficient to no body fat, a fetus may not survive. To prevent this, estrogen signals fat to be laid down in typically female areas (around the hips and bottom), giving women a pear-like shape to better serve the childbirth process.

During menstruating years the ovaries make estrogen, although small amounts are produced by the fat cells and the adrenal glands. At menopause, ovarian production of hormones ceases.

It is estrogen that begins breast tissue production at the first signs of puberty. It broadens hips, and gives women their curves. When it is in excess, estrogen unfortunately promotes fluid retention and this in itself can be a very stressful thing for a female. Her clothes don't fit her the way she would like them to, and if she is feeling this way it can impact on a woman's desire to be intimate, which can, for some women, lead to challenges within the significant relationship of their life and adds yet another layer of stress.

Fluid retention

It is not physically possible to gain 7lbs (3kg) of body fat in one day and yet women regularly tell me that this has happened to them.

As I said earlier, I have never once weighed a client and I don't encourage anyone else to do so either. I do this for many reasons, but one is certainly because the amount of fluid being retained is directly correlated to hormone level fluctuations over the month.

Besides, when you weigh yourself, remember that all you are really doing is weighing your self-esteem. I am convinced that many women 'feel' fat when really they are either bloated or retaining fluid. I have met thousands of women who can gain a few pounds in a day, and this messes with their mind in a catastrophic way. If you get on the scales in the morning and weigh 155lbs (70kg), and, by the evening, you weigh 161lbs (73kg), it's easy to feel incredibly disheartened and wonder how on earth this could possibly happen. It doesn't matter if you've eaten well and exercised that day (though it can be harder to comprehend when you have) or if you haven't – it can add an additional layer of stress to an already overloaded female mind... something else to worry over.

The only possible cause of gaining 7lbs (3kg) in one day is fluid retention. Even if a woman is aware of this, the very act of seeing the additional figure on the scale over the course of a day, or even a week, will make the majority feel fat, frustrated, anxious, impatient, and just generally lousy.

And in this state, do you think you are more likely to make good food choices? Do you think you'll feel like being intimate with your partner when you're overly conscious of your fleshy and puffy parts? Do you think you'll be motivated to exercise because if you're still gaining weight even while you're eating well and exercising it must mean you need to exercise even more and when are you going to find the time to do that because you're already struggling to keep up with what you're doing now... and that was all thought in such a hurry that now you are gulping for air!

Fluid retention can be a result of more factors than we can go into here but to give you some idea, it can be created by poor progesterone production, a congested liver, poor lymphatic flow and mineral deficiencies or imbalances.

Awareness

From an energetic medicine perspective, fluid retention can relate to holding on to things that we really need to let go of. Think about who or what you may be holding on to that is no longer of benefit to you. Perhaps it is a belief that no longer serves you, and your body is simply trying to wake you up to this and get you to change.

When it comes to excess fluid, estrogen is another likely culprit. It can also drive headaches, including migraines, increase blood clotting, decrease libido, and interfere with thyroid hormone production and, due to its relationship to progesterone, lead us to feel like we have to do everything with haste – big health consequences all due to too much of one little hormone.

The role of progesterone

We looked at the effect of low progesterone in Chapter 2 (see page 28) so let's look at what role it plays in our sex hormone balance. Reproductively, progesterone is responsible for holding in place the lining of the uterus that estrogen has laid down. In the event that conception takes place, your progesterone levels will continue to rise, as the lining of the uterus needs to be maintained instead of shed. In the event that there is no conception, the lining of the uterus is not needed, so progesterone levels fall away, initiating menstruation. In an optimal sex hormone balance, progesterone is the dominant sex hormone from just after mid-cycle onward until menstruation.

Biologically, progesterone has numerous other roles, all pivotal to the Rushing Woman's Syndrome message. Remember, progesterone is a powerful antianxiety agent, an antidepressant, and a diuretic, and it is essential if you are to access fat reserves to burn for energy. If you don't have the right amounts of progesterone in your body, you will always burn glucose as a fuel and this may result in your body having to break down muscles for energy – even if you have fat reserves there – which will slow your metabolism over time. So, low progesterone may be the source of a tendency to an anxious or depressed mood and, if you feel like you have a blessed life and yet you still feel low or like you complain too much, add guilt to that emotional cocktail and a degree of confusion about what is really bothering you. You can see how layer upon layer of physical and emotional stress can form.

The stress and sex hormones relationship

The relationship between sex hormones and stress hormones is fascinating and powerful, and it's where an aspect of the physical, biochemical approach of Rushing Woman's Syndrome is focused. And this is because nine out of 10 women who see me for consultations enjoy positive changes in their body and their health when we address this.

Estrogen is the dominant sex hormone between days one and 14 of the menstrual cycle. For the first half of the menstrual cycle, a relatively small amount of progesterone is made from our adrenal glands. For the sake of this description, let's call the amount two units.

However, as you now understand from the previous section, your adrenal glands are also where you make your stress hormones, namely adrenalin and cortisol. We've talked about how adrenalin communicates to every cell of your body that your life is being threatened, even though all that may have happened is that you've overslept, been late for work, had a hectic day, and jumped on the scales to see that you're heavier than you were yesterday. My point is to highlight that both physical (e.g. caffeine) and emotional (perception of your weight and urgency through your day) processes drive adrenalin production and communicate danger.

Cortisol, as you now understand, communicates to every cell of your body that there is no food left in the world and, as a result, it wants your body to break muscle down and store fat – even if it's just a result of you being internally rattled.

Since, from your body's perspective, progesterone is intrinsically linked to fertility, if there is a signal going off inside indicating that your life is under threat and that there is no food left in the world, the last thing it wants is for you to conceive so it shuts down production of progesterone in your adrenal glands. This means that both estrogen and cortisol are still signaling to store fat and you've lost the counterbalancing hormone that helps to keep you calm, burns fat, and gets rid of excess fluid.

In my opinion this kind of situation is an enormous shift in female chemistry, quite unique to our modern lifestyle, and it plays havoc on our physical and emotional wellbeing. This is one of the key underlying shifts that creates a perception that you need to rush. We can go from feeling happy, healthy, centered, and energized, with great clarity of mind and an even mood, to having a foggy brain and feeling either overly anxious about things we cannot name or utterly exhausted as a result of this shift to excess estrogen and cortisol coupled with low progesterone. Physically we may feel puffy, heavy, bloated and full of fluid, with a sense that our clothes are getting tighter by the minute. And that is just the first half of the cycle!

During your menstrual years, you reach ovulation at around day 14 of your cycle, and there are numerous hormonal changes that occur to drive it. As ovulation occurs, an egg is released from the ovary leaving a crater on its surface. This crater, called the 'corpus luteum,' is where the bulk of a woman's progesterone is made. Progesterone is designed to peak seven days prior to menstruation (on day 21 of a 28-day cycle) at around 25–40 units.

If conception takes place, progesterone levels begin to climb in order to hold the lining of the uterus in place and, at around week 12 of the pregnancy when the placenta has formed, progesterone levels climb to around 300–400 units.

During pregnancy a woman has the highest level of circulating progesterone but as soon as she has birthed the placenta, her progesterone levels plummet from 350 to zero! Thankfully, birth ignites the production of some other feel-good hormones – oxytocin for example, although they tend to be more short-lived.

In previous times, when a baby was born it was brought into a community or extended family. These days, it's much more common (though not exclusively) that a hospital birth is followed by a mother taking her newborn home and caring for it alone while her partner continues to work in order to pay the bills and the mortgage. If there are challenges in their relationship or challenges due to the needs of other children, financial stress, ill or aging parents, an ill newborn or simply one who won't sleep, the new home environment with baby can be highly stressful.

Another example, something I've heard a thousand times, is when a new mother who made what she thought would be a welcome transition into staying at home with her child from a corporate career (whether temporarily or permanently) begins to second-guess her decision. The guilt and confusion that this stressful scenario brings up can be overwhelming and under these kinds of circumstances, the restoration of adrenal progesterone can become compromised. After all, the body is so busy making stress hormones that it believes it cannot be safe for the new mother to make the fertility-linked progesterone.

Remember, progesterone is one of the most powerful antianxiety and antidepressant substances the body makes. On the other hand, if a woman takes her baby home into an environment where there is support and doesn't feel alone with her new precious bundle – which could simply be due to the mother's attitudes, beliefs and perceptions, or due to actual support from other people – then adrenal progesterone levels are far more likely to be restored, and her chemistry is all the better for it.

If conception does not take place during a menstrual cycle then progesterone levels fall since they aren't required to maintain the lining of the uterus, and a period starts. However, something that is so common today is what is known as 'luteal phase insufficiency.' This is where ovarian progesterone production is poor and a peak of 25 units in the second half of the cycle is not reached. It might be that progesterone is the dominant hormone from days 16 to 18 of the cycle, but it falls away too soon (it is supposed to be dominant from just after mid-cycle at around day 14 until around day 27), and estrogen becomes dominant leading into the menstrual bleed.

This estrogen dominance is the biochemical basis of premenstrual syndrome (PMS), something that most Western women experience at some stage in their lives and can be problematic, both for them and for everyone else around them! PMS can occur because estrogen is dominant for all but two or three days of a 28-day cycle, meaning that progesterone gets no time to rule the roost, and a woman misses out on all its delicious stress-busting, calm-inducing, and fat-burning qualities.

What happens when estrogen is dominant?

We've looked at the effects of low progesterone, so now let's look at what it means to be estrogen dominant in the second half of the menstrual cycle, when progesterone is supposed to be at its peak. Estrogen dominance can be created through a number of mechanisms, including ones that involve the nervous system, the adrenals and the liver. You might recognize that your progesterone–estrogen balance is out of whack if you note the following symptoms:

- Premenstrual migraine

- PMS-like symptoms

- Irregular or excessively heavy periods

- Anxiety and nervousness

- Feeling like you can't get your breath past your heart

The typical symptoms of estrogen dominance (which usually also involves low progesterone – but not always) include:

- Irregular periods or excessive vaginal bleeding

- Bloating/fluid retention

- Breast swelling and/or tenderness

- Decreased libido

- Mood swings, most often irritability, easy to anger, and/or depression

- Weight gain, especially around the abdomen and hips

- Cold hands and feet

- Headaches, particularly premenstrual

- Tendency to yellow-tinged skin

Estrogen dominance is the most common hormonal imbalance I see in menstruating women. The combination of a significant excess of estrogen being made within the female body and increased estrogen in our environment (food and chemicals, such as pesticides), appears to be affecting our endocrine (hormonal) systems in literally life-changing ways.

It is paramount to find out whether you are suffering from symptoms of estrogen dominance due to excess estrogen or significantly low progesterone levels. If it is the latter, it would indicate that either adrenal or ovarian production (or both) of progesterone is poor. In this situation, you may still have optimal estrogen levels (neither too high or too low) yet also have challenges with your body fat and/or periods as a result of low progesterone. The hormones that signal ovulation to occur are made by the pituitary gland so, again, optimal progesterone production is reliant on good communication between the pituitary and the ovaries.

Another common scenario involving an excess of estrogen can be due to excessive environmental exposures, including ingestion of pesticides, use of plastics, the oral contraceptive pill, or hormone replacement therapy (HRT). It is also commonly created as a byproduct of poor estrogen detoxification by the liver, which results in estrogen being recycled through the body. Furthermore, body fat makes estrogen, so the higher the levels of body fat, the higher the estrogen load and the more efficient your liver detoxification pathways need to be to clear old estrogen from the body.

In a nutshell, the liver decides whether to excrete or recycle estrogen. The liver prioritizes what it needs to detoxify and because the body makes estrogen itself, it is not a high priority to clear it from the body. This can lead to a woman having not only this month's estrogen circulating around her body but also last month's and perhaps even previous months'. Even a woman who produces optimal amounts of progesterone cannot produce enough to balance out that much estrogen and all of that recycled estrogen increases a woman's risk for estrogen-sensitive reproductive system cancers, including breast cancer.

An additional estrogen-dominant hormonal picture is a combination of both the descriptions above: poor progesterone production and recycled estrogen. This would be far less common in the West if we took better care of our liver. As I love to say, these things have become common, but they are not normal. Women are not supposed to get PMS. Your period is supposed to just turn up... no extreme mood swings, no pain, no premenstrual migraines... just menstruation.

Healthy breasts

Tragically, breast cancer is the leading cancer killer among women aged 20–59 in high-income-earning countries. This is the exact same population affected by PMS and the perceived need to rush. The link between the two is undeniable, in my opinion. Looking after your precious liver is one of the best steps you can take to ensuring your breast tissue remains healthy.

Our breasts are extremely sensitive to both estrogen and progesterone due to the high quantity of receptors to these hormones present there. We've already discussed how a compromised liver will circulate partially detoxified estrogen back into your blood when it can't keep up with its load.

Many women knowingly or unknowingly regularly drink too much alcohol, and yet research clearly indicates that regular consumption of alcohol is inextricably linked to many cancers,[1-3] including a strong link with breast cancer,[4-6] and some health organizations suggest that there is no safe level of consumption of alcohol for women, and particularly if there is a history of breast cancer. Really contemplate this.

When we couple this with adrenal glands that are prioritizing stress hormone production over sex hormone production, we have a scenario where breast tissue can be readily affected. Progesterone has been shown to be protective against breast cancer (except those that are progesterone-receptor positive) so in many cases balancing out your sex hormones can be a great start to offering protection from breast cancer.

Caffeine – and coffee in particular – has also been found to play a role in the creation of denser, cystic breast tissue.[7] Green tea, on the other hand, has consistently been shown in numerous studies to be protective against many types of cancers, breast cancer included.[8]

Action

Challenge yourself to take a break from alcohol and coffee, no matter how much you love or depend on them. Do it for one week – one small week out of your long life. Once you've managed one, try another. Even better, refrain from both caffeine and alcohol for one or two menstrual cycles and notice how different your breasts feel.

Supporting your breast health with good nutrition

A diet filled with vegetables and fruits also goes a long way to promoting healthy breast tissue. There is a significant body of evidence that a diet based mostly on plants[9] – with a reduction of animal products, fried foods, and charcoal-grilled meats[10-11] – is beneficial to breast health. All vegetables from the Brassica family are rich with anticancer properties.[12-13] Broccoli in particular contains sulforaphane which is a compound that assists your body in the elimination of potentially carcinogenic substances in as little as 10 days after it is included in the diet on a daily basis. It also keeps estrogen from binding to and stimulating the growth of breast cancer cells, a vital step in keeping breast tissue healthy. The great news, too, is that sulforaphane survives cooking.

Fruits and vegetables rich in beta-carotene can also help to protect your breasts. Women with breast cancer tend to have lower levels of beta-carotene in their blood, on average, than women who don't.[14] However, researchers have been unable to identify if this is a cause or result of the disease.

Action

One of the most effective and safest ways to maintain healthy levels of beta-carotene is to consume five or more servings of dark green, orange or yellow vegetables and citrus fruits daily.

There is also a growing body of literature that links insulin resistance to numerous cancers. As a hormone that encourages all cells to grow, fat cells, healthy normal cells as well as cells that may be precancerous or cancerous, it can behave like a growth factor. The best way to limit insulin production in the body is never to base a meal purely on carbohydrates. The only carbs humans traditionally ate were those from berries, legumes, and pulses (we might call these lentils and beans, such as garbanzo beans or chickpeas). Limit your intake of the barrage of highly processed foods rich in sugars and starches that we are currently faced with. Also, don't forget that most alcoholic drinks contain more sugar than you might realize.

Remember, it is what you do every day that will have the most impact on your health, not what you do sometimes. It is not about going without; it is about getting real about what you, as a woman, already know to be true. You know better than anyone when you have too much of a particular substance in your diet... whether it is alcohol, coffee, or sugar. Make the changes you know you need to make now. You will give your breasts a great chance of remaining healthy in the process.

Lastly, the benefits of regular movement are well documented for many areas of our health, including a reduction in insulin levels and body fat, both of which, in excess, have been linked to unhealthy breast tissue.

Action

Regular exercise is great for overall health but there are plenty of simple ways to shift your body out of the sedentary zone. Include a short daily walk in your routine, perhaps during your lunch hour or after dinner; try to park further away from the store or your office and then enjoy a longer walk to work; take the kids to the park after school and play football; or find an exercise app that encourages you to do a workout each day. There are so many ways to increase your activity level; make a plan and action it. Restorative movement is best for those with adrenal fatigue.

There are specific nutrients that are paramount for healthy breasts. While most of us have heard about the importance of iodine for optimal thyroid function and in the prevention of goiter, what we hear very little about is how vital it is for breast health. Both the ovaries and the breasts concentrate iodine and the ovaries can produce a specific form of estrogen that is linked to breast cancer when there is an iodine deficiency.[15-17] Once iodine levels are optimal, this has been shown to be reversible.

To increase your iodine intake use a salt that contains iodine, add seaweeds to cooking, or take a supplement. You only need a small amount each day and you can have too much, so be guided by a health professional about the right amount of iodine for you.

Our dietary intake and ratio of essential fatty acids is also of great consequence to breast health. Essential fatty acids are predominantly found in oily fish, algae, flaxseeds, chia seeds, walnuts, pecans, evening primrose oil, blackcurrant oil, and borage oil. Consuming enough of these vital fats on a daily basis through your diet can be challenging so a good supplement that combines at least fish, algae or flax with evening primrose oil can be highly beneficial. Begin with two capsules both morning and night or one to two tablespoons of a food-based liquid oil.

Magnesium and selenium are also essential minerals for healthy breast tissue and both have been shown to reduce the incidences of new breast cancers. Brazil nuts are rich in selenium and green, leafy vegetables are high in magnesium. Eat them daily, or take a supplement.

When it comes to so many aspects of our health, vitamin C is one of the most important nutrients. Among an endless list of wonderful activities, it helps to keep the immune system responding appropriately to stimuli, and hastens white blood cell response time. Vitamin B6 is another vitamin with extensive research linking it to good breast health. Eggs, bananas and avocados are all good sources.

There are a number of herbs that are also great for breast health. Licorice and peonia are two of my favorites. They support healthy estrogen-to-progesterone ratios (read more about them at www.bioblends.co.nz), while also working on the adrenal glands to help modulate the stress response.

There are also herbs that promote good liver detoxification and bile production from the gallbladder, biochemical reactions that are both essential for healthy breast tissue. Herbs that are useful for this are globe artichoke, bupleurum, schisandra, and St. Mary's thistle. These herbs are best dispensed under the direction of an experienced herbalist.

Reducing your exposure to environmental toxins

In addition to increasing consumption of the above foods, nutrients and herbs, we need to reduce our exposure to those things that interrupt the maintenance and creation of healthy breast tissues. We've already talked about coffee and alcohol; additionally avoiding growth-factor-like substances, including insulin, may be important.

Dairy products naturally contain growth factors, since the milk is designed to grow an 88lb (40kg) baby calf into a 2,000lb (900kg) beast. The growth factors naturally present in milk and milk products drive this growth. Humans, however, aren't designed to grow at these rates. If milk must be consumed, sheep and goats are smaller animals so their milks tend to drive slower, smaller growth rates. Alternatively, plant-based milks contain no growth factors.

There is also a growing and alarming body of evidence suggesting that we need to reduce our exposure to pesticides and plastics. These substances can mimic estrogen and disrupt our endocrine (hormonal) systems. Research in the USA has shown that a growing percentage of girls as young as eight have begun to hit puberty and links poor diet, high body fat, lack of exercise, and an exposure to plastics[18-19] as the likely culprits for the earlier onset of menstruation. We can make a really big difference to our health and our children's health by getting these lifestyle factors on track.

Reproductive system conditions

If an imbalance of sex hormones becomes chronic, there are a number of resulting conditions that can have different effects on how a woman feels and functions.

Polycystic ovarian syndrome (PCOS)

In PCOS, the eggs in the ovaries ripen on the surface of the ovary but are not released. Instead, they harden and form cysts (hence the name of the condition). As you now understand, ovulation is essential to obtain optimal progesterone levels crucial for calm and fat-burning, since the majority of your monthly progesterone is made in your ovaries by the corpus luteum (see page 78).

Other hormones are also involved in PCOS. The pituitary gland makes luteinizing hormone (LH) and follicle stimulating hormone (FSH). Just prior to day 14 of a typical menstrual cycle, both hormones increase, but in PCOS both of these hormones from the pituitary gland tend to flatline, they don't surge to signal ovulation. Testosterone and other androgens also tend to be higher in women with PCOS.

The LH and FSH hormonal profile of an ideal menstrual cycle is illustrated in figure 4 below while the profile of someone with PCOS is represented in figure 5.

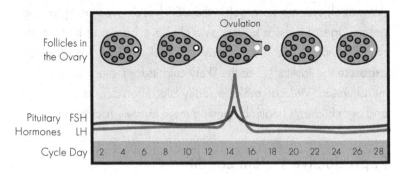

Figure 4: Ideal LH and FSH peaks generating ovulation
Both LH and FSH peak to drive ovulation.

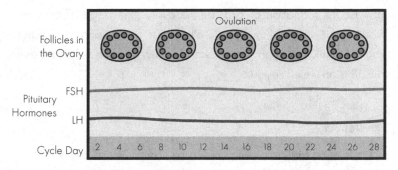

Figure 5: Typical PCOS LH and FSH profile
Both LH and FSH tend to flatline in PCOS, with LH
levels remaining consistently elevated.

Biochemistry, beliefs, and femininity

When it comes to challenges with the reproductive system or hormones, we need to explore not only our biochemistry but also the subconscious beliefs and behaviors, as this is often the gateway to real change and health improvements. And in PCOS I have found this to be absolutely paramount.

When looking at PCOS from a hormonal perspective, not only do the two pituitary hormones, LH and FSH, tend to flatline, but both of the other female sex hormones, estrogen and progesterone, tend to be low. Sometimes estrogen is elevated. Additionally, testosterone tends to be on the high end of normal or elevated out of the normal range. In most other reproductive system health conditions, estrogen tends always to be high. Many researchers have proposed theories about why estrogen tends to be low in PCOS. They include genetics, poor transformation of cholesterol into estrogen and an altered hypothalamic-pituitary-adrenal (HPA) axis, which is the system that links those three glands via hormonal communication. HPA axis function is significantly affected by stress and, in some women with PCOS, it is theorized that a possible outcome of overt or silent stress may be the formation of cysts on the ovary (see page 88). When working with clients, I investigate all of these factors and encourage you to know where you sit biochemically with all of these hormones if PCOS is an issue for you.

Reflect

It is also worth exploring health conditions from an emotional and a metaphysical perspective to help an individual gain more insight into any belief that may be behind the issue.

Think about it from this angle. There is nothing more feminine than our ovaries; men don't have them. With PCOS, however, it is as if the ovaries have gone deaf. The pituitary gland has been calling out to the ovaries in an attempt to alert them to release an egg, the most feminine process that goes on inside a woman. For the ovaries no longer to hear the call from the pituitary, it is possible that there could be a very silent, unconscious belief from somewhere in this person's world that they need to act like a man (or with more masculine behaviors) in order to receive appreciation, connection, or love. Somewhere in their past, more masculine behavior has been rewarded.

Women have shown they can match men in every arena. However, even today there are types of work that are still male dominated. I have met countless women, working in what were previously more male-dominated roles in particular, whose hormonal profiles have taken on a decidedly masculine appearance. These women are incredibly capable. The problem, however, lies in their (usually unconscious) beliefs about how they have to be in order to perform and achieve and, without realizing it, therefore be 'loved.' Most often, they do not even realize that they are thinking or behaving 'like a man' until we explore what that looks like. It is the mental approach to the work not the work or job itself that tends to be masculine.

Please don't misunderstand me. I am in no way suggesting that all professional women have got or will get PCOS. I am also not suggesting that we as women need to behave like men in order to have a highly successful career. What I am simply wanting to point out is that your attitude, your perception of who you have to be, how you must behave, what you have to achieve or do to get approval is likely to be based on more masculine ways. It may not have ever struck you that you even believe certain things about how you have to be, to be loved or to fit in, let alone that there is another way to live.

With our ancient chemistry, we have to respect that what we ask of our bodies today is entirely different from what we asked of them even 100 years ago. On the one hand, it is extraordinary how resilient our bodies can be: we may work 16-hour days sitting at a desk, eat more processed than nutrient-dense food, while we constantly think up solutions to challenges presented during the day, meet deadlines, juggle phone calls, crises, and complaints, and hopefully also celebrate a few things – and despite the pressure this puts on our systems, our body allows us to continue to do it. On the other hand, we are so very far removed from the way humans have lived for 149,900 years that I believe the human body is rebelling, and one of the most obvious areas is women's reproductive health, including fertility.

Action

One of the ways you can counteract this, if it's ringing true for you, is to explore ways that you can bring more feminine rituals into your life. What do you associate with femininity? If your work requires you to be 'masculine,' do it, but bring compassion into your heart and soften your gaze when you're there. No one will know this is what you've done. Instead of tensing up as you look at the work on your desk or in your inbox, notice the work on your desk and take a long slow breath that moves your belly when you inhale, calming and centering you.

Feel, and I mean really feel, really notice what tension feels like in your body. And then relax into it. Only you know you've done this. So many women have become incredibly detached from their body and as a result they are completely unaware of how they truly feel in it. The feminine feels. By relaxing into your body, feeling your tension and letting it dissolve, your productivity and contribution will perhaps be even more than what you found possible from a state of tension. Think about 'creating' instead of 'producing.' In emotional medicine, the ovaries are the seats of creativity. Just that shift in language is more feminine and can be helpful.

When you come home, shift out of work mode into home mode. We play so many different roles these days. Change your clothes. Light a candle and notice the scent. Dance around your house to music that lights you up, if that spins your tires. Later in the evening, have a bath with aromatic oils. Giggle with the children or at a comedy. If it appeals to you, read a book. Make a pot of herbal tea after dinner in your favorite teapot and make it a 'special occasion.' Notice the design of the pot and cup, the fragrance of the tea, and how you feel taking care of yourself. Masculine energy would never do this – but a man embracing his feminine would, just to point out the difference.

Please understand, I'm not suggesting that women are not able to do all of the things men can do – we are just wired differently biochemically. Getting health results, when it comes to PCOS, is all about addressing the biochemistry and cultivating calm in the body. Sharing this with you is in essence, simply a way to highlight the wonderful benefit I have witnessed when women have embraced their feminine essence through more areas of their lives. And rituals that cultivate femininity can be a useful place to begin.

If you're a woman with PCOS I encourage you to explore your perception of your father's expectations of you or who you perceive you had to be to 'earn' his love – you will more than likely see that this is at the heart of why you do much of what you do and that that is OK. Only it is no longer OK if it is hurting your health, which is another reason we are here.

Puberty

Some girls breeze through this time of transition without much change in their moods or their bodies, while for others anxiety or even darkness can set in. Estrogen is the first female sex hormone to be made in any great quantity in our bodies. As beautiful as estrogen can be as a hormone, it can wreak havoc when it is present in substantial amounts for the first time ever in a young female body that doesn't yet have sufficient progesterone to counterbalance its effects.

Prior to menstruation beginning (called 'menarche'), estrogen causes the breasts to bud and promotes the growth of pubic hair. It also begins to drive fat storage and some girls appear to be more 'fleshy' for a time just prior to menarche, indicating estrogen is fulfilling its role.

As you know progesterone is a powerful antianxiety agent and an antidepressant, but if it is slow to initiate, a girl who was once bouncy, bright, full of energy, and interested in things, can become flat or anxious in her moods and distant in her relationships. If her periods do begin and they are irregular and/or heavy and painful, to the extent she is unable cope with school or life in general, she will often be encouraged to take the oral contraceptive pill. It is important to understand two things here. One is the way the contraceptive pills work and the second is the biochemical process that occurs at the onset of menstruation.

First, the pill is successful at preventing pregnancy because it shuts down the ovarian production of hormones. The number of women of all ages who have no idea how this powerful medication works never ceases to astound me. I am neither pro- nor anti-pill; I simply want people to make informed choices. I will say it again. The pill shuts down ovarian production of hormones, and the body relies entirely on the synthetic version of hormones being supplied by the tablet. Substances in patented medications, such as the pill, must be at least 10 percent different from the form the body naturally makes.

With the ovaries shut down, the adrenal production of progesterone becomes even more important, yet is unlikely to be optimal given the onset of menstruation and, for some girls, the increase in body fat for the first time often gives rise to undue stress. For this reason, don't ever comment on an adolescent girl's changing shape and size by encouraging her to eat less. That stresses her more, as she may feel like she is letting you down when she doesn't do it; it doesn't matter whether you are her parent, teacher or friend. Explain that, for a while, hormones can change our shape, and eating nutritious food and staying active are the most important things to do to stay healthy. Tell her not to worry about it and demonstrate your love for her with your actions not just words. With less stress, which may be due to her private perception of how her life is, which may gently be explored, her progesterone is more likely to kick in, and her body shape and size will sort itself out. Some areas that can be useful to explore in this situation are an adolescent female's perception of academic pressure and her perception of what it may mean to a family member if she 'fails' (which may mean not coming out on top of her class in some cases). Exploring what her 'friends' are saying at school can also prove insightful.

The second issue to explore is the biochemistry associated with the onset of menstruation. This is the first time in a girl's life that her pituitary gland sends signals to her ovaries. For approximately the first five years, the chemical messengers released by the pituitary follow a road to the ovaries that looks like a goat track, meaning that it is a path that sometimes reaches a destination (in this case the ovaries) and sometimes winds up heading off into no-man's-land. In other words, sometimes the pituitary signals miss their mark. After about five years, this pathway, if it has been allowed to establish, behaves like a five-lane highway. The route is clear, straight, and unhindered.

However, what I repeatedly see is girls that have gone on to the pill to manage irregular or very heavy periods rather than for contraception, shortly after menstruation begins. If sport is a big issue or school is being missed due to severe period pain, then perhaps there may be occasions when the use of the pill is appropriate, and I certainly do not want to elicit feelings of guilt in parents or daughters in this area. But the pill simply masks the truth. If a girl stays on the pill long-term, the five-lane highway is never established. She will then come off the pill in adulthood, potentially wanting to have babies, but her pituitary has no history of communicating with her ovaries. It is a lot to ask your ovaries to suddenly wake up after suppressing their function for an extended period of time.

I cannot encourage you enough to get to the bottom of why the pain or the irregularity occurs in the first place. Before deciding about whether or not the pill is the best choice, explore other options and seek ways to change the hormonal imbalance that may be present, or at least give the pituitary–ovary pathway time to become established.

As far as moods are concerned, what breaks my heart is seeing a young woman start menstruating, with very heavy periods and some weight gain – despite still eating well – and disappear into her mind with her own private focus on sad thoughts and an anxiety that often comes out with nervous-type behaviors, such as biting or picking her fingernails. This can be the first time ever that a girl experiences a tendency to depression or anxiety, and her family is often bereft and concerned at the change in their girl. The most common intervention in this situation is the prescription of the pill. But because the pill does not correct what is likely to be slow-starting, or insufficient, progesterone, the young woman's mood doesn't lift, despite her periods now being regulated (by the pill). So she is encouraged by well-meaning adults to take an antidepressant. She is not even halfway through her teens, and she is on two incredibly potent, powerful medications.

There are times when conventional medicine is lifesaving, and I am not suggesting it be avoided at all costs – especially not at the cost of precious human life. What I am encouraging, initially, is the balancing of estrogen and progesterone through natural methods with the support of an experienced health professional. Counseling at the same time may also be incredibly beneficial to assist with any new darker thoughts. My holistic approach means also discussing any fears about self-perception of what it means to be an adult woman. Puberty can be the first time that a girl ever feels fleshy, puffy or bloated, and to a young mind – likely influenced heavily by popular magazines – it is easy to understand why she can think she is fat when she is simply estrogen dominant. As I said earlier, it is not physically possible to gain 7lbs (3kg) of fat in one day, and it is most likely due to fluid. And given the diuretic action of progesterone, a deficiency of this vital hormone is one of the likely culprits of this young woman's fleshy feelings.

Menopause

At its simplest level, menopause is the ceasing of the ovarian production of hormones. But production continues from the adrenal glands and fat cells. However, as explained earlier, many women now make insufficient amounts of progesterone from their adrenals because of chronic stress. In my opinion, this is such a powerful factor in whether a woman breezes through menopause with few or no debilitating symptoms, or whether the heat and the sleeplessness become overwhelming. If you are approaching menopause, I cannot encourage you enough to ensure your adrenal function is optimal.

Action

If menopause is in sight or underway, then apply the adrenal care techniques described in Chapters 4 and 11 (see pages 65 and 218), and use breathing strategies and herbal support, combined with lifestyle changes where possible.

If you are postmenopausal, I also can't encourage you enough to address adrenal health and liver health, strategies for which are also in the solutions section. Heat from the body can certainly be due to low estrogen levels or liver congestion. If a client describes having tried all sorts of natural estrogen therapies and used herbs that have an estrogenic action such as black cohosh, and they are still overwhelmingly hot and suffering debilitating hot flashes (also known as 'flushes'), I will usually treat their liver.

Remember that in traditional circles, menopause is a time when wisdom begins to flow constantly. Trust what you already know inside of you when it comes to your health. You innately know better than anyone else what is best for you. Seek guidance from health professionals, but apply what makes sense to you.

Menstruation and rest

Many women already know what I am about to share with you. Perhaps this is something you have observed in yourself and that is, that menstruation can be a time of soothing, stilling calm, a natural bliss. With some care and attention from you, this time can become your own natural, inbuilt zone to de-stress.

In our 24/7 lifestyles it is more important than ever to create islands of calm; timeout when we can release tension and simply 'be' for a while. Just as we can't go without sleep for too long, your psyche cannot push on for too long without some quality downtime. The time you menstruate is the classic cyclic downtime due to the hormonal pattern and the energetics that exists at that time. The hormone involved is called oxytocin, also known as the love hormone, as it engenders feelings of love, calm, and belonging. It is released during sexual activity, birth and breastfeeding, as well as when we are touching, hugging, and sharing a meal. Orgasm causes oxytocin levels to rise from three to five times higher than baseline, creating feelings of closeness and tenderness after lovemaking. Oxytocin is also released at menstruation as the uterus contracts at this time of the cycle.

For so many women today, however, the lead-up to their period is a source of great despair, pain, misery, temper outbursts, and tears. Yet even with these states of upset (which I want so much for you to be relieved of; please follow the advice in the solutions section, as you do not need to put up with menstrual cycle challenges!) if you were to pause, you would notice that a calm state is available to you at this time.

In the West we have an epidemic of exhaustion. We push and push and push and don't allow ourselves enough downtime. There are very few women in the Western world who would not benefit enormously from more rest. For women, menstruation is the natural time for this and as a bonus during this time, an innate 'natural calm' is on offer. Lifestyle changes may need to be made, however, to be able to soak up what is on offer at this time.

Action

Slow down as you come into and during menstruation. Go to bed earlier. Apart from getting good-quality rest, there is evidence that the extra dreaming time is good for easing PMS. Sleep is the all-round number one remedy, and it is free.

One of the strategies I suggest is to keep track of your menstrual period and reduce your commitments in the lead-up to and during that time, particularly on day one of bleeding. Even if you have to go to work, do your best not to push yourself too hard that day. If what you've just read makes you roll your eyes and exclaim on the inside that I clearly have no idea what your life is like, take a breath. There are very few women in the West who don't have 60 million things on their plate. But every minute of every day you choose how to spend your time. Granted it may not be possible every single month to give yourself the gift of some downtime during menstruation, but do everything in your power to make this happen. Your body's innate wisdom guides you to do this so let it be your guide more often. Even just doing this, I've seen women have far more regular, less challenging menstruation.

If you have PCOS and don't menstruate, schedule your downtime for the first night of the dark moon. Science and history teach us that the ovaries are stimulated by light. Historically, before electric light, women tended to ovulate on the full moon and bleed on the dark moon.

Action

The effect of moonlight is beneficial to your body so take the time to look at the moon as often as you can. If you have to go outside at night, don't just tend to the dog or run to your car, look up at the night sky and notice the moon. I encourage you to draw her silver light into your ovaries and imagine them being lit up. This is a particularly important exercise if you don't menstruate regularly. While you do this be sure to breathe diaphragmatically. Combined with attention to diet and herbs, this very feminine ritual can be incredibly beneficial to menstrual cycle health and calm.

Scientific research supports the need for more quiet time.[20] A day of absolute solitude was found to be the best antidote for what were shown to be 'overtaxed, overstuffed brains' and the ideal way to attain optimal brain performance. Another researcher claimed that 'everyone in the study was chronically stimulated, socially and physically, and we are probably operating at a stimulation level higher than that for which our species evolved.' This scientist's remedy was to spend more time alone. Two other scientists also found that attentive listening to silence helps the human brain to focus, while what has been coined 'conscious menstruation' by brilliant authors Jane Bennett and Alexandra Pope, has also been found to be a way to attain optimal brain performance.

Slowing down and becoming more conscious is crucial to our wellbeing. If we ignore our need to 'chillax' (as my best friend's son says when he needs to chill out and relax all at once) or withdraw during menstruation, it may contribute to the development of some of the classic PMS symptoms, such as disorientation, dreaminess, fogginess, overwhelm and irritability, as well as headaches and menstrual pain. However, if you can see your period as a time to turn down the volume, take a break, or perhaps just do less, the calm on offer will find you.

One of my clients who insists on going to the gym seven days a week decided to walk in nature instead on the days of her period to see if that helped. It has and she has now embraced this new ritual. Another lady got her closest friends together and asked them all to share their menstruation dates. They all plugged the dates into their phones and they make a point of getting in touch on the day their friends' periods are due to see if there is anything they can do to help out such as minding their children for an hour or so that day. Gorgeous. Women are amazing.

Even if you lead a very high-pressured life with barely a moment to yourself, with just a simple change in attitude you can start to get a taste of the natural calm on offer to you at the time of your period.

Action

The next time it is day one of your cycle take a moment before you race (hopefully not!) into your day and notice how your body feels to you. Just acknowledge whatever you notice. Wonder to yourself – if you didn't have to work or worry about others today, what would you most love to do? Then, with curiosity rather than despair, drama or frustration, consider how you might give yourself 20 minutes of that on that day.

When I've asked women what they most love to do, the majority reply that they would love nothing better than simply curling up with a great book or a pile of magazines and not having to worry about anything or anyone. So ladies, please, examine your schedule and be ruthless about cutting out what is not essential on the first day of your period, even 'fun' things like catching up with a friend for lunch.

Notice how you might leak energy by getting caught up in drama, gossip, or having to listen to other people's problems. Do your best to excuse yourself from these situations as quickly as you can, for this is the one day you need to receive. Do your best to eat well on this day too. At first simply become aware of this pattern in your month. The more aware of this cycle and this opportunity for calm you become, the more you will feel like you can make little changes that will open this stage up for you and the more effective you are also likely to be in your professional life. Renewal and rest are crucial to our health. You now need to allow it.

Menstruation and menopause are feminine and very natural processes. They offer incredible insight into your general health, as well as a window into your inner world of subconscious thoughts and beliefs. These thoughts and beliefs drive so much of what you do and how you feel. They can be a barometer guiding you to remember what you were born knowing – that you are the embodiment of loveliness.

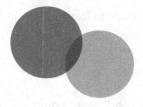

Chapter 6

Hormonal Havoc Part III: Metabolic Mayhem

The Impact of Rush on Your Thyroid Hormones

When it comes to feeling the rush, the thyroid gland is another part of the endocrine system that both contributes to and is affected by our environment and our perceptions. And again, the pituitary gland, in this case influenced by the hypothalamus, controls thyroid function. Understanding where any dysfunction may have come from and the mechanisms involved is crucial to improving your health, your body size and how you feel on a daily basis.

The thyroid gland is a little butterfly-shaped gland that sits in your throat area. This part of your endocrine system is responsible for making hormones that play an enormous role in regulating your metabolic rate along with your temperature and energy. I have met countless people in my working life who show me blood test results that demonstrate that everything is in the 'normal range' and yet who exhibit virtually every symptom of an underactive thyroid. More on 'normal' ranges later. First, here are some symptoms that your body may present you with to let you know that your thyroid needs investigation and/or support.

If underactive:

- You have 'unexplained' weight gain.

- You feel cold in your bones; or you notice you are colder than others around you – you are the first to put on a sweater.

- When you read symptoms of an underactive thyroid, they resonate with you yet you are told your blood test results are fine; when you see them, though, they tend to be skewed to one end of the 'normal' range.

- You have a tendency toward constipation.

- You have long-term estrogen dominance symptoms e.g. PMS.

- You feel weary to your bones; you are beyond tired. Your body feels heavy and lethargic.

- Your reactions to stimuli – both physical and emotional – feel slow.

- You crave salt.

- You crave coffee and it doesn't amp you up – your brain feels slightly more functional after you have it.

- You get groin aches.

- Your voice has changed; it is husky on occasions, particularly when you are extra tired (can also be a sign that the adrenals need support).

- You feel like you retain fluid.

- You have a tendency to a depressed mood, forgetfulness and a sense of being easily confused.

- You experience hair loss.

- You have brittle hair and nails.

- You have dry skin.

- You are having difficulty conceiving.

- You have challenges with menstruation.

- You experience recurrent headaches.

- You've had your gallbladder removed.

- You suffer with chronic stress.

- You have a family history of poor thyroid function or disease.

- You have a family history of autoimmune conditions.

- You have been diagnosed with adrenal fatigue or another condition involving the endocrine system; or you have been previously diagnosed with an autoimmune condition.

- You wonder when it will be your turn; when will you be able to do what you want to do, rather than what others want or need from you.

If overactive:

- You have 'unexplained' weight loss.

- You overheat easily.

- You have a tendency toward 'unexplained' loose stools.

- You experience rapid heartbeat or heart palpitations.

- Your regularly feel amped up and tend toward anxious feelings.

- Your eyes bulge forward from the eye sockets.

- You have chronic stress.

- You have a family history of thyroid dysfunction or disease.

- You have a family history of autoimmune conditions.

- You have been diagnosed with adrenal fatigue or another condition involving the endocrine system; or you have been previously diagnosed with an autoimmune condition.

Please note that many of the symptoms of an overactive thyroid are often the opposite of an underactive thyroid; some people may experience both conditions in their lifetime.

Thyroid hormones

Thyroid hormones are produced as a result of a cascade of signals from different glands, as well as the thyroid gland. This means that if you have a problem with thyroid hormone levels, or with debilitating symptoms indicating something is awry with your thyroid function, then it is essential to get to the heart of the matter so treatment can be appropriately targeted.

The hormone cascade begins in the hypothalamus, in a gland that sends a signal to another tiny gland that sits at the base of your brain called the pituitary gland, which we've already seen also produces hormones involved in menstruation. This signal tells the pituitary gland to make a hormone called thyroid-stimulating hormone (TSH) and then this hormone signals the thyroid to make one if its hormones known simply as T4 (thyroxin). T4 is found in the blood in two forms, namely T4 and free T4 (FT4). They are the same hormone, except one is 'free' to enter tissues and the other is bound up and unable to enter tissues, which is where the work needs to be done. However, both T4 and FT4 are inactive hormones, and must be converted into the active thyroid hormone called T3 (tri-iodothyronine). It is T3 that drives your metabolic rate and capacity to burn body fat. Figure 6, opposite, illustrates the hormonal cascade.

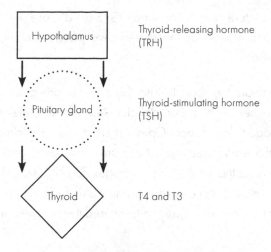

Figure 6: The thyroid hormone cascade
Signaling begins with the hypothalamus communicating with the pituitary gland, which then in turn signals the thyroid gland to make its hormones.

For our body to produce an optimum level of thyroid hormones, a number of nutrients are essential. Two minerals that are vital to this process of conversion that literally lights up your metabolic rate are selenium and iodine. Since the majority of soil in the Western world no longer contains these trace minerals, they cannot be in the food that is grown in them and so many people today get very little in their diets.

There are two scenarios that are associated with the thyroid gland – it can become overactive, which is known as hyperthyroidism, or underactive, which is known as hypothyroidism. The latter scenario is the one that can lead to weight gain that can be challenging to shift until the underlying thyroid issue is addressed. For some people, swinging between an underactive and an overactive thyroid occurs. This vital gland is also susceptible to autoimmune diseases, which is where your immune system begins to see the thyroid gland as a foreign particle like a germ. It then attacks it, leading to a change in its function that can end up in either the overactive picture (this is known as Graves' disease with the autoimmune involvement) or the underactive picture (known as Hashimoto's thyroiditis).

Other major factors that can initiate this process are poor liver function, iodine, selenium or iron deficiencies, infection, elevated cortisol or estrogen dominance. Consider what you have already learned from the earlier sections about stress hormones and sex hormones and read that list again (see pages 70–72). It is behind the 'why' where most of the answers lie and it is therefore important to work out which path led someone to altered thyroid function.

Hypothyroidism: Underactive thyroid gland function

One of the first things that springs to mind with underactive thyroid people is that they almost always tell me that coffee makes them happy and the first 20 minutes or so after they've had a coffee, is the only time they feel what they call 'normal.' A 'thyroid person' will also usually tell me that chocolate helps them, and if they feel this way, it is potentially not just the caffeine content of the chocolate but it may also be due to the dopamine-enhancing actions of this food. Dopamine is a neurotransmitter that when in low supply can be involved in depression, while too much can drive addictive behaviors. For someone with poor thyroid function, chocolate may give them a little lift. Please don't necessarily assume that if you love chocolate you are a 'thyroid person' – many people simply love chocolate.

The classic symptoms of hypothyroidism are listed above but if your thyroid gland is underactive, you're likely to feel deeply fatigued and more depressed in mood than racy and anxious. However, I've met countless women who, from a mood and behavior perspective, appear to bounce between these two extremes, so it is important to explore both the under- and overactive thyroid health pictures. And given that the thyroid is controlled by the pituitary, when the whole endocrine system is not able to work optimally due to your perception of pressure and a lack of 'safety' in your world, the thyroid is a likely target for dysfunction.

Let's explore the roads to an underactive thyroid and where to begin to support your thyroid health.

Infection and poor liver detoxification

Common roads to hypothyroidism are a history of Epstein-Barr virus, also known as glandular fever and mononucleosis (at any stage of life) and liver overload, or a congested liver, as I sometimes refer to it. To treat both of these roads requires prioritizing care of the liver. You'll find liver-love strategies in Chapter 11 (see page 230). Also, an excellent herb to use if you have a background of chronic infection (and if a herbalist agrees that it meets your needs) is astragalus.

Mineral deficiencies

We've already touched on how hypothyroidism can be influenced by iron, iodine and selenium deficiencies so choose foods that are rich in these minerals. Use Celtic sea salt with iodine and/or cook with seaweeds such as Kombu. Good food sources of iron include beef, lamb, eggs, mussels, sardines, lentils, green leafy vegetables, and dates. There is a small amount of iron in many foods, so eating a varied diet is important. And remember that absorption is enhanced by vitamin C. Don't assume that if you're vegetarian or vegan you are iron deficient – some bodies utilize the iron from vegetable sources very efficiently.

> **Action**
>
> You can check both your iron and your iron storage (ferritin) levels with a blood test.

The other option is to take a supplement that covers these nutrients. There are some excellent thyroid support capsules on the market so seek out one of these if it appeals. Regarding iron, it is wise to have a test before you supplement, as overloading your liver with it can be problematic (although this is uncommon). On the other hand, if you are deficient, without supplementation it will be a very slow and challenging process to get your iron levels back up. Many iron supplements are constipating, but most people find this doesn't happen with liquid iron supplements.

Iodine is a trace mineral that is essential to health. Without iodine, the thyroid gland is unable to make thyroid hormones. Iodine is also essential to the IQ of the developing brain in utero and studies are now showing that some children in the West are suffering from such low iodine levels that their IQ is being detrimentally affected.

We used to get iodine from salt – it was first iodized in the USA in 1924 – and, apart from the anticaking agent that is usually added to it, there's nothing much wrong with it. However with the advent of rock and Celtic sea salts, iodized salt is no longer so popular and means that many of us are simply not getting enough iodine. Food sources of iodine include all seaweeds (e.g. nori). Iodine is found in small amounts in seafood, but even eating seafood every day will not provide you with adequate amounts of iodine

Iodine is also a difficult mineral to test for, as accurate tests require you to collect 24 hours of urine and, remarkably, not all countries offer this testing. Adult females require 120µg (micrograms) and males require 150μg of iodine per day to prevent deficiency. It is far more beneficial, however, to individualize doses. I have known of cases where amounts between 12–50mg (milligrams) are initially necessary to treat a deficient state, and this can be easily done with one to three drops of a good-quality liquid iodine solution per day, available from some health food shops or through a compounding pharmacist. It is best to obtain specific advice to learn how to meet your individual needs and because you can have too much iodine, this must be guided by a health professional.

Estrogen dominance

Thyroid function can be suppressed by too much estrogen. Conversely, optimal progesterone levels support its function. Apply the strategies for dealing with estrogen dominance outlined in Chapter 5, if you suspect that this is the basis for your challenge with your thyroid gland.

Elevated cortisol due to stress

Stress due to elevated cortisol interferes with the production of the active, fat-burning thyroid hormone T3, slowing down your metabolism. Additionally, your body is urged to break down muscle to provide glucose for your brain (as already covered) and muscle reduction also slows down your metabolic rate. In the absence of stress, a healthy body converts FT4 into T3, but with elevated cortisol levels, the conversion of FT4 to T3 decreases. This diminished function of conversion also occurs if you restrict your food intake. Your body doesn't understand that you may be trying to drop body fat and simply follows its overarching goal of survival, slowing down your metabolic rate to preserve those precious fat stores.

Elevated cortisol also inhibits the release of TSH from the pituitary and with less TSH, the body produces less FT4. Apply the strategies for high cortisol outlined in Chapter 4, if this scenario rings true for you. Elevated cholesterol can also be a result of poor thyroid function and once thyroid function has been treated, cholesterol returns to normal (if it is not the result of a congested liver).

Thyroid medications

Typically, if you have been diagnosed with an underactive thyroid, you will be prescribed thyroxin (T4). While on this medication, some people feel brilliant and it resolves all of their hypothyroid symptoms, including weight gain. If you're someone who is on this medication (and has been for a while) and have not found you've experienced good results, try a different approach. Thyroxin will not suddenly start to work after years of taking it, if it has not done so yet. (You must never cease taking thyroid medication without the guidance of an experienced medical professional.) If you want to stick with conventional medicine, tell your general practitioner you feel lousy on your current medication (if you do) and that you would like to try a different drug. There are numerous brands of thyroxin on the market. Sometimes a thyroid medication that is subsidized shifts to a different brand and I have had hundreds of clients who were happily taking one form of thyroxin only to find some of their symptoms return when they take the new brand. It sounds odd, yes, but the body doesn't lie. Explore this even if your blood levels of TSH, FT4, and T3 are 'normal,' but you still have symptoms.

In my opinion, an excellent option to try when it comes to hypothyroidism is whole thyroid extract (WTE). This is taken instead of any synthetic medication and, unlike the synthetics providing only one of the thyroid hormones, WTE provides all of the thyroid hormones. This product is made by a compounding pharmacist and it is essential that if you wish to be guided in the transition from a synthetic to the WTE that you speak with your doctor about it.

If you exhibit numerous symptoms but have not been diagnosed with a thyroid illness, do not rely solely on your blood tests to determine if your thyroid is underactive. Work with a health professional who will treat the symptoms, not just the blood, and will monitor both your symptoms and the blood work as you explore treatments.

Thyroid antibodies

An autoimmune response occurs when the immune system mounts an immune response against the tissues of the body, rather than a germ. If this occurs, it is measurable in the blood, as antibody levels specific for particular cell or tissue types can be assessed. This can occur in many parts of the body, including the thyroid. Unfortunately, autoimmune thyroid diseases are increasing, particularly among women in the West. If you have an underactive thyroid (measured by hormone levels) with antibodies, this is known as Hashimoto's thyroiditis. If you have an overactive thyroid with antibodies, it is called Graves' disease.

Health professionals are typically taught that if someone has thyroid hormone levels inside the 'normal' range, they won't have antibodies and that the only time testing thyroid auto-antibodies is warranted is if hormone levels are outside the normal range. Yet I have found time and time again that this is not the case. I have assisted countless clients to find a thyroid problem that is behind their tired but wired feeling, body-fat changes, unexpected body-temperature alterations, anxious feelings, unexplained inability to conceive (to name a few symptoms) who have 'normal' thyroid hormone levels and sky-high antibody levels.

If you present with many of the symptoms of an over- or underactive thyroid, yet your hormone tests are normal, in my experience it is worth testing thyroid antibodies as this can shed light on what really needs attention.

Hyperthyroidism: Overactive thyroid gland function

Common signs and symptoms of an overactive thyroid are listed on page 105. Thyroid hormones have a direct effect on most organs, including the heart, which beats faster and harder under the influence of thyroid hormones. Essentially, all cells in the body will respond to increased thyroid hormone levels with an increase in the rate at which they conduct their business.

When it comes to an overactive thyroid, whether there is autoimmune involvement (Graves' disease) or not, a frantic pace of life has been involved with every single case I have worked with. In my experience, stress, specifically the pace of life and what each woman has demanded of her body, is the major factor in the development of hyperthyroidism. More than any other group, they have sacrificed sleep and they have juggled more in their lives to date than most people could juggle in a lifetime. As I like to say to one of my favorite rushing friends, 'it is as if you run a small country' with all that she handles. And there is usually a part of them that actually quite enjoys life this way. They are often at a bit of a loss as to why their body has gone and done this to them (presented with elevated anti-thyroid antibodies along with elevated thyroid hormone function tests).

Yet their body has sent them a powerful message that the way they were living was not serving their health or perhaps even their destiny and what life had in store for them. I believe that your body does its best to wake you up to pay attention to what really needs your attention, every day. I've seen some overactive thyroid conditions return to normal with this acknowledgment and the subsequent lifestyle change that must go with it. All of the women I've worked with who have successfully returned their thyroid function to normal (from being overactive), and had a complete remission of their symptoms, have literally changed their lives. Quite often they change their jobs, or if that's not an option for them, instead they change their attitude and approach to that work and their life in general, completely. It has been an inspiration to witness this in my clients. Louise Hay suggests in her wonderful book, *You Can Heal Your Life*, that on a metaphysical level there may be a feeling of 'rage at being left out,' and she encourages people to affirm, 'I am the center of my life, and I approve of myself and all that I see.'

When your body is getting the message that it needs to speed everything up, it is virtually impossible to slow down and approach life from a calm, centered space. When your heart feels as though it might jump out of your chest, it can be practically impossible to join a meditation class. So the physical aspect of this condition most certainly needs to be sorted out. However, I want to encourage you also to get to the real reason of why you may have run your life at such an intense pace in the first place. The whys are explored later in Chapter 9.

Blood tests and 'normal' ranges

We have a 'normal' range in blood testing to provide a cutoff that helps to indicate when something may be abnormal. We need these ranges to guide us. It would be chaotic without them. I have great concerns, however, when we base the future of a person's health on blood tests alone.

According to Dr. Karen Coates – an insightful and pioneering general practitioner and coauthor of *Embracing The Warrior: An Essential Guide for Women* – the normal range for some blood tests is calculated periodically by each pathology laboratory to ensure that the reference range printed on the test results is 'accurate.' They do this by collecting the first 100 blood samples and testing them for their (in this case) TSH levels – this then determines the reference range. Or it might be progesterone or estrogen levels as another example. But if you think about it, people don't usually have blood tests because they are feeling fantastic – most often it's the opposite. And yet, we seemingly base our 'normal' ranges on these figures.

Furthermore, it is also important to understand how the 'average' amount of a particular nutrient or hormone is calculated. Mathematically, the top reference point is calculated to be 'two standard deviations' above the average, while the bottom figure is 'two standard deviations' below the average. The arbitrary rules of this method dictate that 95 percent of the 100 blood samples taken must fall into the 'normal' range. The statistical definition of standard deviations insists that only four or five results may fall outside this reference range, two samples below and two above.

When taking in this information, there are two important points to consider. Firstly, the reference ranges for some blood parameters are getting broader. When I wrote the first draft of my first book *Accidentally Overweight*, the normal range for TSH was 0.4 to 4.0. Four months later, by the time the book was ready to go to publication, the normal range had shifted to 0.3 to 5.0.

People at either end of this 'normal' spectrum are unlikely to be feeling as though their thyroid is functioning optimally and will more than likely be exhibiting thyroid symptoms. If they are symptom-free, it means their body is not trying to draw their attention to the thyroid gland and it's not a problem. However, my concern is this: if we base treatment on the blood work alone and leave people to live with their symptoms with their result skewed to one end of the normal range, we are risking, not optimizing, their health and overall wellbeing, not to mention their quality and enjoyment of life. This brings me to my next point, which is, given the 'normal' range is based on individuals who are potentially unwell, this process is somewhat flawed from the start. It is more challenging to create optimal health, prevent disease, and maximize quality of life for people when they are being guided with their blood tests to fall into a potentially unhealthy normal range.

Your blood tests

If you have blood tests done by your doctor, I urge you to get copies of your own blood tests and look for results being skewed to one end of the normal range. Let me explain.

Where I currently reside, the normal range for TSH is 0.5 to 5.0. Those numbers may seem small but someone with a TSH of 0.5 will typically feel and look completely different to a person who has a TSH of 5. Also take into account that if your results happen to fall within the normal range you will usually be told by well-meaning professionals that there is no problem with your thyroid. I have often seen a TSH (made by the pituitary) blood result of 2.5 or greater in a person when their body was screaming out to the thyroid gland to make FT4. Normal FT4 levels sit somewhere between 10–20 and regularly I see someone experiencing symptoms of hypothyroidism with an FT4 of 11. This person feels exhausted in their bones, has trouble naturally using their bowels daily, has dry skin, very low motivation, a tendency to a depressed mood, brain fog, and their clothes are gradually getting tighter. Their thyroid needs support.

In cases such as these, starting with iodine and selenium is always my first port of call, and sometimes iron too, is part of the first step. Additionally, working to support the adrenals, resolve estrogen dominance if it is present, switch to a grain-free diet, and getting real about your beliefs and your perception of what life is like for you can all work its magic on normalizing the thyroid.

Louise Hay, the brilliant metaphysical medicine pioneer, teaches that thyroid problems represent feelings and beliefs around humiliation and feeling like you never get to do what you want to do (how many mothers – in particular – does that describe?). Louise Hay suggests someone with thyroid problems unconsciously asks, 'When is it going to be my turn?' She suggests you develop a new thought pattern of 'I move beyond old limitations and now allow myself to express freely and creatively.' Underneath diagnosed hypothyroidism, Louise Hay suggests, are feelings of hopelessness, a feeling of being stifled, and a sense of giving up. She suggests you develop a new thought pattern of 'I create a new life with new rules that totally support me.'

I include this so as to provide you with a complete picture of your thyroid health: from conventional function of glands and hormones, why you need to be aware not to rely solely on your blood tests, what the thyroid needs nutritionally through to the metaphysical. Somewhere among these three approaches lies your answer, not necessarily in one or the other. I urge you to explore all three.

Action

If you exhibit the symptoms of your thyroid not working properly – whether it be overactive or underactive – despite blood tests being normal, please work with a health professional who will treat your body (the symptoms) and use blood results as a guide, rather than solely relying on blood tests. If your thyroid is at the heart of why you feel tired but wired, why your body-fat levels have changed despite nothing else really changing, why you feel anxious for no reason you can identify or why you haven't been able to conceive, then supporting its function can offer you such an enhanced quality of life.

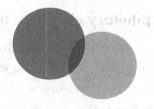

Chapter 7
Hormonal Havoc Part IV: The Mother Gland

The Impact of Rush on Your Pituitary Gland

I always aim to get to the heart of the health matter with clients. This usually involves exploring what is happening for them physically and emotionally. There are numerous body systems intricately involved in our physical and emotional health, how we look, how we feel, and how we behave. And as you have just read, as well as the nervous system, the endocrine system holds the key to so much about how we feel. After the hypothalamus, the master control center for our hormonal systems is the pituitary gland, a gland that is often overlooked when exploring women's health unless symptoms distinctively point to a problem in this area. Yet creating an environment inside the body that allows the pituitary gland to work optimally can be the key to nullifying the panic as well as regulating all of the other endocrine glands including the adrenals, the ovaries, and the thyroid.

What does the pituitary gland control?

The pituitary gland is a pea-sized gland located at the base of the skull between the optic nerves, and its main task is to secrete hormones. The reason the pituitary is sometimes referred to as the 'master gland' is that it controls hormone functions such as our temperature, thyroid activity, growth during childhood, urine production, and ovulation. In effect the gland functions as a thermostat, controlling all other glands that are responsible for hormone secretion. The gland is a critical part of our ability to respond to the environment most often without our knowledge. It is the link between our nervous system and our endocrine systems. Figure 7 below shows the location of the pituitary gland, housed in the brain about level with the bridge of your nose, and the glands it affects.

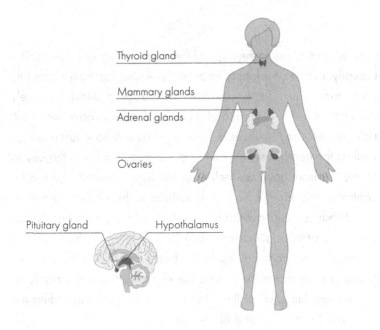

Figure 7: The role of the pituitary gland
The pituitary controls many aspects of the endocrine system by sending messages to other glands to make more or fewer hormones.

The pituitary gland actually functions as two separate compartments: an anterior (front) portion and the posterior (back) portion. The anterior gland is made up of a separate collection of individual cells that act as distinct factories, termed 'functional units,' which are dedicated to producing a specific regulatory hormone messenger or factor. These factors are secreted in response to the outside environment and the internal bodily responses to this environment. These pituitary factors then travel into the bloodstream and eventually reach their specific target gland. There they stimulate the gland to produce the appropriate type and amount of hormone so the body can respond to the environment correctly. Isn't that amazing in itself?

There are 'factories' for a number of specific hormones, including a cortisol factory, for growth hormone, prolactin (related mostly to lactation), gonadotropin (stimulates the gonads), and another for thyroid-related stimulation. These five factories function as the anterior pituitary gland neuroendocrine unit. Again, no need to worry about any of these long-winded scientific names, I simply want you to see that the pituitary plays the role of the master controller of the endocrine glands we have explored in the previous sections.

The posterior part of the pituitary stores and secretes hormones made by the hypothalamus. Both sections of the pituitary are directly connected to, and controlled by, the hypothalamus, a section of the brain controlling the basic survival processes of hunger, thirst, sexual reproduction, and self-defense. A stem containing both neurons (the nervous system) and small blood vessels (to transport the hormones of the endocrine system) connects the pituitary gland with the hypothalamus. Therefore, the hypothalamus communicates with the pituitary in two ways: by nerve impulses and by chemical messengers (hormones). The anterior pituitary receives instructions from the hypothalamus in the form of releasing hormones. These chemical messengers produced by the hypothalamus then travel through the blood. A special network of vessels directs this blood through the anterior pituitary. In contrast, the posterior pituitary receives its messages through neural tissue and is controlled by nerve impulses.

If any one of the factories in the anterior part of the pituitary becomes excited and starts to overproduce their respective hormonal factor, the net result is excess production of the final hormone product. For example, if the cortisol cells, called corticotrophs, lose their ability to respond to the normal stimuli from the environment and from the hypothalamus and develop their own independent, uncontrolled autonomous secretion, they will produce more cortisol than the body requires. In return the adrenal glands will be overstimulated and secrete unregulated and unneeded stress chemicals, called 'catecholamines.' The net result is excess production of these important chemicals, which can signal fat storage, affect blood pressure (usually elevate it), and drive the heart rate higher, among other things. This can cause the body and internal organs to be stressed when there is no need.

Unfortunately, the consequences of overdriving the internal organs of the body can take a toll on your health and, eventually, be life threatening. In extreme, and rare, cases, the cells that overproduce their respective hormones can clump together within a given area of the pituitary gland creating a true factory of overproduction, which would be diagnosed as a pituitary tumor. Not all pituitary tumors are cancerous; however, all tumors need medical attention due to the hormonal dysregulation they promote.

The pituitary gland makes six hormones from the front part of the gland and two from the back. The front part makes:

- Thyroid Stimulating Hormone (TSH), which signals the thyroid gland to make thyroid hormones
- Luteinizing Hormone (LH), which signals the ovaries

- Follicle Stimulating Hormone (FSH)

- Prolactin, which stimulates breast development and breast milk production

- Growth hormone for the growth of all tissues in the body

- Adrenocorticotrophic hormone (ACTH), which signals to the adrenals to make cortisone (which is converted into cortisol)

The back part makes:

- Antidiuretic hormone (ADH), which controls how much urine is passed

- Oxytocin, which signals the uterus to contract at appropriate times in life (e.g. during childbirth and orgasm)

There are other endocrine glands in the body that do not need the pituitary gland to give them messages to produce their hormones. These glands include the parathyroids for calcium regulation and the pancreas for insulin production. They are controlled through other mechanisms.

To give you an example of how one of these pituitary hormones works, let's look at ACTH, whose job it is to direct the adrenal glands, whose function is essential to life. The hypothalamus produces an ACTH-releasing factor that stimulates ACTH secretion from the pituitary into the bloodstream. Specifically programmed receptors on the adrenal glands pick up the ACTH and these receptors start sending signals to the nucleus, or center, of the cells to start producing and secreting adrenal hormones. These hormones are then released into the circulatory system and their presence is communicated to the brain. The broad (family) names for some of these hormones include the glucocorticoids (such as cortisol, see Chapter 4, page 47), which influences the metabolism of the body, the mineralocorticoids (such as aldosterone), which are involved in regulating the amount of water in the body and hence blood pressure; and progesterone (see Chapter 2, page 28).

Like so many other hormones, ACTH is secreted in a circadian pattern over a 24-hour period. Each individual has their own internal circadian rhythm, which determines how much sleep they need, when they are most alert, and when they prefer to eat. Disruptions of this rhythm can affect biological functions and moods, as well as intellectual ability. For example, jetlag is probably the result of a disruption of the circadian rhythm.

For most people, ACTH is at its highest blood level in the early morning and, with its action on the adrenals and the subsequent hormones that are produced, it influences whether you bound or crawl out of bed, and because the adrenals are the place from which we make our stress hormones, it seems, over time, that if the stress goes on for too long, they become less able to adapt to our surroundings. In other words, they are getting the message that they need to make stress hormones when you may, in fact, be safe.

Obvious symptoms of pituitary problems

When there is significant dysfunction with the pituitary gland (please note, this is rare), the following symptoms are common:

- Headaches
- Visual disturbances
- Fatigue and lethargy
- Unexpected abnormal growth
- Sleep disturbance
- Nipple discharge
- Impotence (men)

- Absence or disturbance of the menstrual cycle

- Skin and hair changes

Not everyone will experience all of these symptoms at once or even at all. These signs and symptoms may occur because the target organ is not working effectively, it may not be the 'fault' of the pituitary gland itself. There are tests an endocrinologist can run to determine what precisely is going on. When there is a diagnosed pituitary condition, it will usually be necessary for an endocrinologist to prescribe the hormones to be replaced.

Suboptimal pituitary function (no disease)

I have seen countless women display symptoms that involve all or most of the organs the pituitary governs without them having a full-blown pituitary condition. I call this 'suboptimal pituitary function.'

These women will display symptoms involving the adrenal glands (related to stress hormones), often the reproductive system (e.g. PMS, PCOS, endometriosis, debilitating menopause), and sometimes the thyroid. If these women read information on the Internet they will tell me they can't work out if their problem is their adrenals, their sex hormones, or their thyroid, as they relate to all the symptoms of dysfunction for each gland (see pages 14–15, 70–72, and 104–106). They are usually tired but wired and rarely sleep well. Their moods change easily and unpredictably and they are often impatient with the people they love the most in this world. And then berate themselves for being this way... hardly a winning formula for a happy life. If it is not clear to me based on the symptoms, I will test the stress hormones, the sex hormones, and thyroid function to get a clearer picture. And what has become apparent to me is that for so many women today, all three of these systems are affected and not only do each of the affected glands need support, the pituitary does too.

I believe that this is the result of subconscious fear, which is at the heart of why we rush. As we will explore in the emotions section, this fear can be due to real threat or perceived 'threat.' I meet countless women who tell me that they are in love. And they are! And yet they are also in fear... fear that they won't do a good enough job, fear that they are not there enough for their children, fear their intimate relationship will end unless they are a certain way, fear that they will go broke, fear that they will get yelled at... and so they do everything in their power to avoid ever having to feel that they are not enough because it instinctively triggers the switch that they won't be loved... remember Chapter 1 (see page 8.) To prevent their fears from becoming realities, they go into overdrive, which, for some women, appears to take its toll on the pituitary gland and the glands it controls.

Control

Here's the 'weirdo medicine' aspect of how I consider health conditions... if the pituitary gland is the control center for the human body, then it seems logical to conclude that this gland will be particularly affected in women who describe themselves as 'control freaks,' women who have forgotten how to trust the unfolding of life, that it is all part of a bigger picture that we can't often see or understand, and they've forgotten to be present in every moment.

I was reminded recently of the joy we can, as adults, so easily miss. I was sitting on a park bench, watching people from all walks of life enjoy the sunshine and outdoors. A mother threw a ball to her two sons (ages eight and ten), one of whom had a developmental delay. He didn't catch the ball every time she threw it to him while her other son did. When the developmentally typical boy caught the ball, he had no change of expression on his face, or in his manner, and he simply threw the ball back to his mother. The boy with the developmental delay, however, celebrated every time he caught it! The delight and the excitement every time he caught the ball was as amped up as the first time he caught it, and he literally jumped with joy every time before he threw it back to his mother. Catching the ball had become routine to the younger, developmentally typical child, and he had lost his connection of glee to his ability, while the developmentally delayed child was truly living in the moment and outwardly demonstrating how thrilled he was with his achievement every time it happened.

Reflect

How many of your skills do you take for granted and no longer notice? Do you still pause at the feeling of human contact, someone else's skin on yours? Or the feeling of your pet's fur under your fingertips? Do you pause and breathe and tune in to how this feels? It is ultimately feminine to feel. The first time you felt these things, it would have felt like magic to you. Pause long enough in each moment to experience the magic. It is on offer 24/7. But when we take our life for granted and tune out, and when we rush, we go momentarily blind. It is time to live your life in the light again and allow your pituitary gland to flourish.

Am I 'safe'?

The typical health picture I am witnessing in more and more women is as follows. The hypothalamus asks the question 'am I safe?' 24/7. It has always done this. In doing so, it is assessing your physical environment – i.e. is it too hot, too cold? – and also emotionally. The trouble is, we have beliefs that we don't even know we have. We create meanings from the looks on people's faces and the things they say, based on what we experienced as a child, whether we realize this or not. The way we think the world is, isn't how it really is. We tell ourselves stories constantly about who we are and who and what we have to be to be safe and loved. And, if based on the meanings we have set up in the nervous system, the hypothalamus perceives that we are not safe (from being yelled at or 'criticized', for example) then, without us knowing, it sends a message to the pituitary gland, which fires off the SNS and all of the necessary hormones so we are ready to fight or flee.

That means the adrenals make adrenalin and/or cortisol and most often both. The adrenal production of progesterone is therefore decreased, meaning we lose this vital antianxiety agent, and estrogen becomes dominant, which makes us fleshy, puffy, and kind of crazy. This means the thyroid gets a signal to either amp up or decrease its hormone production, and blood glucose is not astutely regulated, which can lead us to feel like we want to eat an arm off. All of the above makes it harder and harder to sleep well, further setting us up, biochemically, to rush. The 'not feeling safe' feeds the cycle. And the chemistry the cycle elicits keeps it going.

But when I spell it out like that, you can see where you may need to start – with your own mind. Of course I will offer you solutions for the various hormonal pictures I've just described in the coming chapters – that is a huge part of what I do and why women's health improves – and of course I will encourage you to step up and do all you can to give your body the opportunity it is screaming out for to balance your sex hormones and stop churning out stress hormones, and reinvigorate your thyroid. There is much you can do to assist your body to do this. Yet at the same time, if I don't strongly urge you literally to get to the heart of the matter, and see why you rush, why you don't feel 'safe,' it is like trying to stop a bath from overflowing by easing the plug out of the hole to allow a small amount of water to escape.

Exploring the emotional side of your health allows you to turn off the tap. Real food fosters that exploration, that enquiry. One of my key messages is this: It is very difficult to be kind, compassionate, and patient with others when you are filling yourself with stimulants and food that contains very little nutritional value. Choose real food that nourishes you, and watch your physical as well as your emotional health shine.

So all I want for you right now at this stage in the book is recognize the body systems that may need support. Don't worry about how you are going to do that right now. Just recognize, with immense compassion for yourself, that it is what it is. And the power to change your health is in your hands. And I achingly want to assist you.

The intense stress of natural disasters and world unrest

There have tragically been many disasters in the world of late (across all times sadly), both natural (such as earthquakes) and domestic (such as violence), and unspeakable acts of violence globally. And when I talk about stress, I certainly do not want to make light of anything any of us may have been through. A natural disaster promotes the fight-or-flight response for a very good reason – to help you get out of danger and save your life. I know for many thousands of women I have met who have been through these events that the stress internally continues long after the events themselves may have passed. I admire your courage and resilience. And I also offer you this statement: The impact and meaning of a catastrophe are not in the event itself. The ability to tolerate it is a function not of what has occurred but of our relationship to ourselves and our own minds. In the simplicity of that realization is freedom.

Humans have an extraordinary resilience, both mentally and physically, and the body has an innate capacity to heal. Remember that! We really are amazing. However, to assist that process, there is much we can do to support our body's stress response. Here, I describe the physicality of the stress response not so you worry more but so that if your body, health, or mind-set start to change, you can rest assured that it is a natural process and that your body has an extraordinary capacity to heal.

Stage 1

Adrenalin, the hormone that makes our heart race, is our acute stress hormone. It is what makes us jump when we are startled, makes us shaky after an acutely stressful incident (such as a car accident) and it drives our thoughts to race. It does all of this, as its primary function is to give us the fuel we need to get out of the life-threatening danger it believes we are in. Since digestion is not a life-saving process, adrenalin stops digestion from working optimally, as it wants you to be ready to deal with whatever is threatening your life. Adrenalin puts us on 'red alert' so that we are geared to fight or flee. Initially, when we get a shock, this is the survival response of the body designed to get us out of danger.

This is the primary stress hormone that will have been made by anyone involved in, or directly affected by, any kind of natural disaster or act of violence. Some people get biochemically stuck in this state because the fear of another event or concerns for family continue psychologically. Since your body perceives that your life is in danger, it won't want you to sleep too deeply in case it stops you from being able to fight or flee the danger, so your sleep can also be affected. The best tactic on the planet to calm yourself from this state is to change your focus to something for which you are grateful (and I don't say that flippantly) and shift your breathing back into a pattern that makes your belly move in and out with each breath, rather than your chest. As we've already discussed, nothing communicates to your nervous system that you are safe better than diaphragmatic breathing (see Chapter 4, page 65).

> **Action**
>
> Taking withania, passionflower, and zizyphus have all been shown to be helpful in dealing with shock. Keeping hydrated is also essential, as is additional vitamin B (found in whole grains), vitamin C (found in many fruits and capsicum), and magnesium (found in green leafy vegetables and nuts).

Stage 2

After the initial shock, the second stage of stress is typically initiated and the body begins to produce cortisol. We've already talked about how cortisol signals to the body to store fat because it believes that there is food scarcity in the world (see Chapter 4, page 51). This may mean you will find yourself regularly eating too much because your cortisol-fuelled body thinks you are so lucky to have found a whole pack of rice crackers!

You will likely find your sleep affected in this stage too. A little different to adrenalin-affected sleep, you probably won't find it too hard to fall asleep but you'll generally wake up between 2 a.m. and 3 a.m., as cortisol naturally rises. Cortisol initially does wonderful things for the body in this state of stress, as it is a powerful anti-inflammatory. We need the anti-inflammatory action to protect us from the inflammation adrenalin can cause. It becomes problematic for our health when the stress goes on too long for our body to handle (this is different for everyone). Plus now you also have cortisol breaking down your muscles to burn as glucose, suppressing your immune system, and giving you an almost uncontrollably sweet tooth.

> **Action**
>
> Excellent ways to support yourself through a period of elevated cortisol include doing your breathing exercises daily, using herbs such as Siberian ginseng, rhodiola, licorice, or withania, and filling your diet with as many fresh foods as you can.

Stage 3

The next biochemical stage of stress that can occur, especially if the stress has been prolonged, may involve cortisol falling low. This is when our body hits 'burnout' or adrenal fatigue, as it is now commonly known. We now know that cortisol is supposed to be high in the morning and it plays a key role in how vital you feel as you get out of bed. Stiffness is a key symptom of adrenal fatigue. For those with chronic stress, morning cortisol levels tend to be low and it can be very difficult to get out of bed with such low levels. By mid-afternoon, they will be at an all-time low, and you feel you need something sweet, something containing caffeine, or a nap to get you through your afternoon.

> **Action**
>
> Deep, deep fatigue can be treated with a herbal tonic that contains panex ginseng, licorice, and astragalus. I almost always also add another herb or two, depending on what else is going for the individual; typically a digestion/liver herb, such as gentian, or a reproductive herb, such as shatavari or peonia. Although I often recommend supplements of herbs and/or nutrients during times of stress, never underestimate the healing and restorative power

of food the way it comes in nature. Taking supplements is not a reason to eat a poor-quality, low-nutrient diet. I simply recommend supplements where appropriate and particularly to assist in the restoration of health. To that end I have created a range of food (plant)-based nutritional supplements called Bio Blends. You can read about their benefits at www.bioblends.co.nz

Finally, human kindness goes such a long way toward healing and we have been privileged to witness such extraordinary acts of courage by so many of the people in our world.

Feeling safe is the key

Pituitary diseases are rare. What is much more common is the pituitary receiving the message that you are not safe and it makes hormones in response to this information. As a result, too many women then suffer the effects of a pituitary gland that is on red alert, almost 24/7, a state we are not designed to live well in. Consider this as you are faced with choices across your day, as your health is ultimately the result of hundreds if not thousands of decisions you make each day. Every thought, food and beverage choice is either leading you toward better health or taking away from that. Ensure that you are making more choices toward true wellness, rather than constantly making withdrawals from your health bank account.

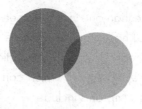

Chapter 8

Digestive Dilemmas

The Impact of Rush on Your Bowels

I am endlessly amazed by how clever and extraordinary our bodies are. It astounds me how many processes happen within our bodies without us having to think about them. One of those incredible processes is digestion. Good digestions provides us with the extraordinary gift of nourishment, which we need in order to survive. Digestion is the process through which we extract all of the goodness from our food. It is intricate and complex but still relatively robust, and it is intimately connected to how you feel and function every single day. It affects everything from the energy you have to the fat you burn, from the texture and appearance of your skin to whether you have a bloated tummy or not.

In fact, digestion impacts everything, right down to your mood. It is the cornerstone for so much that goes on inside us. If you regularly experience digestive complaints, such as reflux, intermittent constipation and diarrhea, or simply just being bloated every evening, it can feel as though this is just how it's always going to be. It must just be how you're built, in your genetics, your lot in life. Well, hear this: bowel challenges do not have to be your reality.

Unfortunately for more than one in five women in the West, irritable bowel syndrome (IBS) has become the bane of their life. They do not have a bowel disease but rather a functional disorder of the digestive system, the symptoms of which can range from mild to debilitating. The main symptoms include:

- Diarrhea or constipation and/or intermittent bouts of both

- Excessive flatulence

- Mucus in the stools

- Bloated abdomen

I know I see a biased group of the population in my practice, but nine out of every 10 women who see me about their health say yes, when I ask them if they have a bloated stomach. Food is not supposed to bloat you.

Before I thoroughly explain IBS and offer you specific advice about what to do about it, it is crucial that you first understand how your digestive system works, as you may identify aspects of what you are experiencing with your tummy along the way. It is also important that you understand more about your digestive system, as it can be a challenge to sort your stress hormone production. For example, 80 percent of the body's total serotonin is in the gut, and as serotonin is our primary happy, calm, content hormone, gut dysfunction can enormously affect our mood.

You may think that some of the following advice is too simple or too obvious but the reality is, we don't always have to make complex changes to make a true difference. The impact of rushing, stress, and urgency, whether you display it in your behavior or hold it all in, on your digestion can be so powerful. So reflect on your own eating habits and digestive system functions as you read on, and be ready to resolve any frustrations you have with your digestive system.

Signs your digestive system needs support include:

- Experiencing reflux and/or indigestion.

- Recurring bad breath and/or bad taste in your mouth.

- You experience recurring diarrhea or constipation, fecal impaction, intermittent bouts of diarrhea and constipation, incomplete evacuation of the bowel, or unpredictable bowel habits.

- You experience bloated, abdominal distension.

- You have excessive wind (based on your perception) and/or offensive odor to flatulence.

- You pass pale, black, frothy, or poorly formed stools (ideally stools look like a sausage) or there is food visible in the stools.

- Gut pain (all gut pain needs to be investigated by your doctor first).

- If you have travelled and had diarrhea (and this has ceased) but you haven't felt the same since.

- Your tummy makes noises and you can hear them, particularly at night.

- You have unexplained fatigue (and other causes have been ruled out).

- You feel lousy/worse after eating.

- You regularly overeat or lose your appetite.

- You belch a lot; even water makes you burp sometimes.

- You have a food sensitivity and are becoming more sensitive to foods.

- You feel stressed regularly.

- You rarely feel hungry (and this is not due to overeating).

- You feel full very quickly.

- You have addictions to some foods.

- You regularly take medication.

- You have taken antibiotics many times.

- You tend toward a low mood.

- You have been diagnosed with depression (remember 80 percent of the body's serotonin is made in the gut; also remember that serotonin is only one of many neurotransmitters potentially involved in low mood).

- Your skin is congested, breaks out easily and unpredictably, or tends toward redness/inflammation.

How the digestive system works

Put simply, digestion is the process through which food is broken down into smaller and smaller components. As an example, proteins are broken down into amino acids so that we can absorb them and use them for energy and nourishment. This ongoing cascade of events sustains our life and it is truly amazing.

The digestive system is made up of a digestive tract – a big long tube (imagine it looking like a hose) – and numerous ancillary organs, including the liver, gallbladder, and pancreas. The tube begins at your mouth, where the digestion process begins with chewing. Food then moves down the esophagus, through a valve, and into your stomach. It then travels through another valve at the bottom end of the stomach and into the small intestine, through the small intestine and ileocecal valve into the large intestine, and finally any waste is excreted out the other end. When our digestion is functioning optimally and this process runs smoothly, you look and feel amazing. If any part of it is compromised, the opposite can be true and it can literally change your life when you resolve your symptoms.

Chew your food

We place food into our mouth and then it moves down the esophagus and into the stomach. But before it reaches the stomach, what do we do to it? Hopefully we chew it rather than inhale it! Since we don't have teeth anywhere other than our mouth, we are obviously unable to chew our food further once we swallow it. Yet so many people eat as though their esophagus is lined with teeth. Eating has been something that many of us do on the run or in between other appointments or activities. If we are particularly struck by the food's flavor we might chew it four times, if we are lucky. It's often a case of chew, chew, chew, chew mmm mmm yum, next forkful in, chew, chew, oh gosh my mouth is so full, better swallow some food... So we swallow some partially chewed food – and some food that hasn't been chewed at all – and we do this day in, day out, year after year. Often we aren't even aware that we do so. And somehow we expect our stomach to cope.

In the end, of course, your stomach gets to a point where it doesn't like the rushing rules by which you are playing. It has no time to prepare itself for the influx of food with the production of stomach acid and digestive enzymes. And given that all of the hormones (for example, adrenalin) and the messages being communicated by your nervous system (sympathetic nervous system activation) are telling your body that your life is in danger, you have no resources available to digest food. Your body believes it needs to fight or run rather than rest and digest.

It is so important to slow down when you eat. If you find this challenging and are a food inhaler, try this: put food into your mouth, chew it really well, and then swallow it before you put the next mouthful in. It can help to put your knife and fork down in between bites (if you're eating something that needs cutlery) or engage in conversation if you're dining with others to help slow down the consumption of food. Or think of your own technique to slow yourself down if you shovel your food in. I know that sounds simple, but try it. It can take an enormous amount of concentration for food inhalers to change their eating behaviors. You need to pay attention when you eat to how you eat and in my ideal world you would only eat in a calm environment. I appreciate this is not always possible but if this is an area you want to work on, do all you can to eat in calm surroundings. It may also be helpful to avoid watching TV, scrolling through your phone or reading while you're eating as all of these are distractions from the digestive process.

Keep an eye on portion size

After you've swallowed your food, the first place it lands is in your stomach. Clench your fist and look at it. That is how big your stomach is without any food in it. Tiny, isn't it? If you're someone who piles your plate high in the evening and inhales a big mountain of food, think about how you're asking your stomach to stretch to accommodate it. For the next 30 minutes minimum, your food sits here so that stomach acid and other digestive juices can really begin to break down the food. It makes sense then that eating too much total food can lead to a bloated stomach and digestive system problems.

> **Awareness**
>
> A rough guide to the amount of food you need to eat at each meal is approximately two fist sizes of concentrated food, such as proteins or carbohydrates. You can, and need to, add as many greens (non-starchy vegetables and/or salad) to that as you like, since they have a very high nutrient content and they are also mostly water.

There are countless people out there that know their portion sizes are too big or that they need to stop eating more food after dinner, yet no matter how hard they try, they can't seem to eat less or stop eating once they start. It always comes back to the why.

Stomach acid is a good thing

When it comes to great digestion, stomach acid is a necessity. The production of this begins before food even arrives in your stomach. Even just the aroma of food before you take a bite can stimulate the production of stomach acid. Its role is to break food down. Imagine your food is a big long string of circles as shown in the first row of figure 8 below. It is the job of the stomach acid to go chop, chop, chop and break the circles apart into smaller bunches, as the second row illustrates.

OOOOOOOOOOOOOOOOOOOOOOOO
↓ (stomach acid) ↓
OOO OO OOO OOO OO OOOO OO

Figure 8: Digestion
*The action of stomach acid on whole foods breaks
them down into their smaller components.*

Your body is governed by pH ranges – the concentration of hydrogen ions present is a measure of acidity or alkalinity. The pH range is based on a scale 0–14, with figures closer to zero being the acid end of the spectrum and 14 being the alkaline end, while 7 is neutral. Every fluid, every tissue, every cell of your body has a pH level at which it performs optimally. For example, the optimal pH of stomach acid is 1.9, which is so acidic it would burn you if it touched your skin. But it won't while it is nicely housed inside your stomach, as the cells that line the stomach itself not only produce stomach acid but are also designed to withstand the super acidic conditions.

There are countless women, and men as well, who have a pH level of stomach acid that is not acidic enough. A pH far greater than the optimal 1.9 will not be ideal for good digestion.

Reflux and indigestion

It is generally assumed by most adults with indigestion or reflux that the burning sensation they experience with heartburn is a result of having too much stomach acid, when generally speaking it is most commonly the opposite. They are usually not making enough stomach acid and/or the pH of it is too high.

Stomach acid is vital in breaking down those circles. If the stomach acid level in our stomach is much higher than 1.9, it leaves larger, undigested segments that must continue along the rest of the digestive tract intact because the stomach acid cannot effectively break the circles apart. Rather than allowing that food to proceed down into the small intestine for the next part of its journey, the body regurgitates the food in an attempt to get rid of it. You then experience the acid burn and assume it is too acidic when in fact it can't break the food down sufficiently to allow it to pass into the small intestine because it is not acidic enough. That 'burn' you feel is simply due to the acid pH being too acidic for the tissue it's exposed to outside of the stomach. So long as the acid is contained in the pouch of the stomach all is well but the moment it escapes out of this area and into areas that are not designed to cope with much level of acidity at all, it creates a problem.

The lining of the esophagus and the first part of the small intestine are the two areas that are typically affected. Many people with reflux respond very well to the stimulation of stomach acid and/or to omitting foods that are a problem for them and experience much fewer symptoms as a result. I have met countless people whose reflux symptoms completely resolved after omitting either dairy products (precisely omitting the casein) and/or gluten, a protein found in the grains wheat, rye, barley, triticale, and oats (although oats are better tolerated by some people). Incredibly, a number of these people had experienced such severe reflux in the past that they had surgery in an attempt to resolve it. When this didn't work, they believed nothing would ever relieve it, not even medication. They were beyond thrilled when dietary change solved it. Not just alleviated it a little. Resolved it.

Awareness

Pay attention to your body after you eat to help you determine what foods make you feel good and which ones your body tells you don't serve you. Your body has wisdom far beyond your mind. It knows better than your taste buds what it wants and what is good for you. And it will let you know this if you choose to pay attention.

I meet people who describe specific foods affecting their reflux but not every time they consume them, and granted this can be a little more of a challenge to solve. However, with this health scenario, it seems to be the combination of the aggravating food with the hormonal and nervous-system scenarios communicating to the body that they need to be on red alert rather than digesting food. I'll get to this in a moment as this same combination can present as the symptoms for IBS or simply a bloated abdomen.

How to get your stomach acid going

The preparation of our meals historically used to be conducted over a much longer period of time. This allowed time for the aromas of the upcoming meal to signal to the stomach that food was on its way. We also alert our brain to send a signal to the stomach letting it know that food is on its way by chewing. Though of course, when we inhale our food (eat quickly), this doesn't happen. The following solutions will also promote healthy digestion.

Apple cider vinegar and lemon juice

You can physically stimulate the production of stomach acid by taking apple cider vinegar and lemon juice, as both promote good stomach acid production. If either of these is new to you, you may prefer to dilute them initially and, ideally, consume them 5–20 minutes before breakfast (or all of your main meals if that appeals). For example, you might begin with half a teaspoon of apple cider vinegar in as much water as you like. As you begin to get accustomed to the taste, gradually increase the proportion of apple cider vinegar (up to around a tablespoon) while simultaneously decreasing the amount of water. If lemon is your preference, start with the juice of half a lemon diluted with warm water to your taste, and then gradually work up to having the juice of a whole lemon in less warm water. (As an aside, it is a good idea to brush your teeth after your meals when you use lemon in order to prevent any potential problems with tooth enamel. Dentists usually suggest waiting 30 minutes after eating to allow the tooth enamel to firm up again.) Use these tips to wake your stomach acid up before you eat.

Avoid water with meals

Water has a pH of 7 – neutral pH – or greater, depending on the mineral content (higher mineral content makes the water more alkaline). We've already discussed that the ideal pH for your stomach is about 1.9, as this promotes the most effective digestion to promote optimal nourishment and also helps to prevent bloating. So what do you think might occur when you add a liquid with a pH of 7 or greater to your stomach acid? You dilute it. To get the maximum nourishment from our food and the best out of ourselves we need all the digestive fire we can muster! So, in an ideal world, don't drink water 30 minutes either side of eating. Aim to drink water between meals, not with them. It can be a challenging habit to break. Set yourself a goal of not drinking with meals for one week, and then try to keep the new habit going. Or add a squeeze of fresh lemon juice if you insist on water with your meal.

pH Levels in your digestive system

Once food has been partially broken down in the stomach, it moves into the beginning of the small intestine via the pyloric sphincter, a one-way valve leading into the duodenum. You'll find this valve in the middle of your chest or just slightly to the left, just below your bra line.

While the food is sitting in your stomach, your pancreas is being sent messages to get ready to secrete sodium bicarbonate, which has a highly alkaline pH, as well as digestive enzymes. This secretion is designed to protect the lining of the first part of the small intestine and also to allow digestion to continue. What is known as a 'pH gradient' is established all the way along the digestive tract, and each region of the big, long tube has an ideal pH. If the pH gradient is not established in the stomach, in other words, if the pH there is higher than ideal, it can create digestion problems further along the tract. These may be symptoms of the small or large intestine, such as bloating, pain, or excessive gas. A less than ideal pH gradient means that the absorption of nutrients may be compromised as well. Digestive symptoms such as a burning sensation underneath the stomach in the valve area described above can also be the result of insufficient pancreatic bicarbonate production. Pain in this area might also indicate that the gallbladder needs some support or investigation. It is best to consult with your health-care professional about this if you feel discomfort in this area.

The key to letting the pancreas know it needs to jump to action and produce bicarbonate and digestive enzymes is to have stomach-acid production at an optimal pH. Our brain sends off a cascade of signals to each part of the digestive system from one organ to the next. Use the strategies I've suggested, especially chewing food well, to stimulate the pancreas to fulfill its role.

There have been occasions when I have suggested clients use supplements of pancreatic enzymes. If there is a genuine lack of enzymes rather than simply poor stomach-acid conditions for a multitude of reasons, this is an appropriate course of action. I usually suggest the strategies before trialing supplements; however, when symptoms are severe and once other causes have been ruled out, a gastroenterologist may measure pancreatic enzyme levels.

Absorbing the goodness

The vast majority of the nutrients in your food are absorbed via the small intestine. Think about that. Your body draws all of the goodness, all of those nutrients into your blood so your body is able to put those nutrients to work doing all of the life-sustaining jobs that they do. Alcohol and vitamin B12 are virtually the only substances you absorb directly out of your stomach (rather than your small intestine) into your blood. Alcohol tends to be in your blood within five minutes of consuming it, which is why people may get tipsy if they drink it on an empty stomach.

Digestive enzymes are secreted, not only from the pancreas but also from the lining of the small intestine, as food moves through the small bowel. These enzymes continue to break down the food we have eaten into its smallest and most basic components.

However, we can't assume that just because we eat something, we get all of the goodness out of it. The absorption of nutrients is reliant on myriad factors – some of which have been discussed above (like inhaling your food, drinking water with your meals or having poor stomach-acid production) – and some of which are discussed shortly. If a food contains, for example, 10mg of magnesium, it's unlikely that you will absorb the whole amount when you eat it. Throw poor digestion into the mix and it's likely you may absorb very little of the goodness from your food. Think that through: nutrients are essential for life and simply as a result of the way you are eating, let alone the foods you might be choosing, you might be robbing yourself of some of the goodness your food provides. Give yourself the best opportunity to absorb as much goodness out of your food as possible by applying the tips above! It may add energy to your years and years to your life.

Gut bacteria can be your friends – and your enemies

Once the food leaves your small intestine, it progresses on to the large intestine. In this area live millions (or possibly trillions) of bacteria. An adult will, on average, have 4–9lbs (2–4kg) of bacteria in their colon. Just as an aside, remember the next time you weigh yourself, that gut bacteria, which are essential for your life, are contributing somewhere between two to four kilos of the number you see on the scale. Can you see how crazy it is to weigh yourself?

Some of the bacteria in your large bowel (colon) are good guys and some are bad guys. Obviously, you want more good guys than bad guys. These gut bacteria are set the task of fermenting whatever you give them. To bring back the circle analogy, gut bugs love it when they receive something that is one or even two circles in size – they know exactly what to do with that. But if the gut bacteria in your colon are presented with fragments of food that are five or even seven circles in size, as a result of a previous digestive process that has not been completed sufficiently, the only thing they can do with it is what they know – ferment it.

The result of fermentation, of course, is gas. Bacterial action on a food source drives the production of gas during fermentation. The health of the cells that line our gut rely on some of those gases. Others seem to cause a bloated, uncomfortable stomach as the day progresses as they irritate the gut – regardless of whether we have eaten 'healthily' or not.

For so many women, a bloated stomach messes with their brain. Looking down and seeing a swollen tummy somehow immediately silently communicates that they are fat, internally to all of the cells in their body. Even feeling as though they have eaten with their health in mind, many of my clients go up a size around the waist as the day progresses. This occurrence can add a layer of stress to our lives that we just don't need. It is especially stressful because they can't fathom why it is happening. Sometimes it is the foods we choose. Sometimes it is the bugs that live in the colon. Sometimes it is because of poor digestion further up the process such as insufficient stomach-acid production. In Traditional Chinese medicine (TCM), this is considered a spleen and/or liver picture and a TCM practitioner is likely to use acupuncture and/or herbs to support these organs. In metaphysical medicine, there is something in your world that you cannot 'digest' and there is a fear that you are yet to resolve.

How stress plays havoc with your digestion

Stress is a major contributing factor when it comes to poor digestion, a bloated tummy, or IBS.

While it might not seem like it as you are experiencing the symptoms of digestive complaints, the body has your best interests at heart. When you are making adrenalin, your body interprets that there is a danger from which you either need to flee or have the energy to fight (see Chapter 2, page 16). Under these circumstances, it doesn't want you to recall that you haven't eaten for a few hours since that's hardly important compared to whatever is threatening your life. And to power your escape your blood supply is diverted away from your digestive system to your arms and your legs. When you are fight-or-flight response too often (SNS dominance) and food arrives, your body doesn't have the resources to digest it. Your rest-and-digest (PNS) governs this vital work.

So if you have been diagnosed with IBS or have a constantly bloated tummy (and have had bowel diseases ruled out) and have not cracked it by attempting every dietary change under the sun properly (and I say 'properly' because I meet countless women who tell me they have cut out dairy, for example, but continued taking milk in their daily cup of coffee...this isn't a proper dairy-free diet!) and you have used herbs to resolve any potential gut bacteria/parasite problem and you still have your symptoms, then I encourage you to see your digestive system symptoms as a wake-up call. This is your body crying out for you to treat yourself differently. What area do you need to focus on? How you eat, drink, move, think, breathe, believe or perceive? It is time to honor the gut feelings you have and trust your intuition. This is a journey from your head to your heart. It is time to stop running (literally and figuratively) and remember that you are not your past, you are not your stories, and that it, whatever it is, can no longer hurt you unless you allow that. It is time to appreciate fully that you are wonderful and that you are loved, just the way you are.

Leaky gut?

There is another concept within digestive health that can have wide-ranging effects on how we feel and function. This fascinating area impacts gut transit time (how quickly food moves through the digestive system), concentration, mood, behavior, and potentially, food addictions. This concept is known as increased gut permeability, or more colloquially 'leaky gut'.

The cells lining a healthy small intestine look like a row of neatly stacked bricks with finger-like projections (called 'villi') side by side, as demonstrated in figure 9 below.

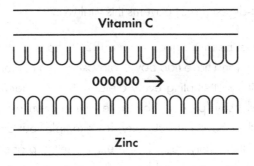

Figure 9: A healthy gut
Food (circles) traveling through a healthy mature intestine move straight ahead. Only nutrients (e.g. vitamin C and zinc) enter the blood vessels that closely follow the intestines.

In a gut with healthy villi, only the tiny nutrients (vitamins and minerals) diffuse (move) through the gut wall into the blood, and it is this process that nourishes us. In a gut that isn't so healthy, the cells lining the gut can begin to space out, as if the bricks are stacked with gaps, as shown in figure 10 below. This is, in fact, how we are born.

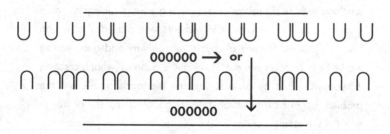

Figure 10: A leaky gut

Microscopic, poorly digested fragments of food (circles) traveling through an immature gut or 'leaky' intestine can escape from the gut and enter the bloodstream.

In adulthood, the cells lining the gut can come apart as a result of the exaggerated production of a protein called 'zonulin' (which we'll explore in more detail shortly), stress or gastrointestinal infection. Since nutrient requirements increase during times of stress, chronic production of stress hormones can signal to gut cells that they need to move further apart so that more nutrition can get through to the blood, compromising the integrity of the entire lining. Everything about us is geared for survival. Trouble is, and as you now understand, we can get stuck in this stress response for many different reasons.

If you have a good cell-lining integrity, as food travels through your gut it can only go straight ahead. In a gut where the cells have come apart, however, it may indeed go straight ahead or it might move across into the bloodstream instead. Unlike vitamins and minerals, food fragments are not intended to enter the blood and so the immune system, thinking the fragment is a germ, mounts a response. And this is one way adults can develop food sensitivities.

Action

If certain foods cause you grief – when once you were able to eat anything without a problem – supporting your gut integrity, while also avoiding some foods or ingredients for a period of time, can heal this process. There's always a reason why and once you've worked out the road into the 'leaky gut' symptoms (what is creating it), you will often be able to tolerate the foods again. Did the problem begin as a result of stress or an infection? The power to heal the symptoms is always in the why, so think about your road in.

Bloating and food addiction

Opioids are substances that help us feel good. They also modulate pain. Endorphins are our natural feel-good hormones and they have an opioid-based structure. If we could literally see the food fragments, we'd see their structure is very similar to that of opioids.

In our brain and gut, we have opioid receptors. When we make endorphins and they bind to the opioid receptors, we feel pleasure. Drugs such as morphine and heroin are opioids and they also bind to these receptors in the brain. Anything that gives a human pleasure has the potential to be addictive, which is why humans can be addicted to these drugs. You can also see how it might be possible for someone to become addicted to exercise since it generates endorphins. So, whatever spins your tires – a sunset, a spin class, a particular fragrance or song, or a child's laughter – what happens in that moment is that you have made endorphins, they have bound to opioid receptors, and you have felt pleasure.

So how is this related to food, rushing, stress and digestion? Some of the fragments of food that can escape out of a leaky gut into the bloodstream can also have an opioid structure. Their names include beta-casomorphine and gluteo-morphine and they are partially digested fragments of casein, the major protein in cow's milk products, and gluten from the grains mentioned earlier. In the exact same way as endorphins, these opioid food structures can very subtly make us feel good by binding to the opioid receptors in our brain. It might not be a noticeable boost in mood but the person will find they have to eat it in some form daily and that they feel they couldn't live without it.

While some women have no problem omitting a food from their diet for a trial period, countless clients have begged me not to take them off a certain food, when they have a set of symptoms that warrants it. This is despite the fact that omitting this particular food for a measly four weeks may just give them the answer to their health concern, There is no judgment here. I simply want to point out the power food can have over us can be akin to an addiction. Our connection to it, our need for it, is often highly emotional and also potentially physical through this opioid mechanism.

Action

If you feel your usual hunger for meals, but as soon as you eat even a small amount, you feel full and possibly bloated, a Traditional Chinese Medicine practitioner would likely suggest stimulating your spleen energy with bitter herbs and acupuncture. Low spleen energy can be a result of what is simply described as overthinking. Within the practice of TCM, relentlessly thinking of what's coming up in your day and an endlessly busy mind take energy away from the vital process of digestion every day. If your liver or kidney (your adrenals, the producers of adrenalin, sit on top of the kidneys) energy is overbearing or low, the spleen may also lose some of its vitality. Working with a wonderful practitioner of TCM can assist you in healing your gut, and many additional digestive system remedies are offered in Chapter 11.

Zonulin and gut integrity

In 2000, a new protein made inside the body was discovered. Named zonulin, it is a physiological modulator of what are called the 'intracellular tight junctions' of the gut. Put simply zonulin plays a role in whether the cells that line the gut are neatly packed together or if they come apart and 'leak.'

Researchers originally thought, for example, that celiac disease, a condition in which gluten drives the immune system to attack the villi that line the small intestine, only involved gluten and genes. What they have since discovered is that zonulin is at a minimum 30 times higher in people with celiac disease, even when they have been on a gluten-free diet for two years, than those without celiac disease – even if they have gut symptoms. What in broad terms can be called 'bad' gut bugs, such as salmonella, have been shown to stimulate zonulin production (which would increase gut permeability/leakiness) and that the presence of these bad bugs enhances gluten's capacity to cause damage to the lining of the intestine; while good bacteria, such as Bifidus bacteria, have been shown to virtually eliminate gluten's ability to cause damage. As an aside, research is currently being done exploring the role of zonulin, increased gut permeability, and the development of autoimmune diseases such as multiple sclerosis and lupus. We'll have to wait and see what the outcomes will be, but I can say for certain that the gut is incredibly crucial to our health.

I include this information here for a few reasons. First, I wanted to highlight that science is constantly teaching us more about the gut and that is a wonderful thing. I believe that in the big scheme of things we know very little about the enormous multitude of roles gut bacteria play in our health. And I wanted to suggest that it is likely that problems with gut bacteria are contributing to the significant increase in gut-based health problems. This is partly, I believe, due to the effect of rushing, as I've outlined above, with the cascade of hormone and nervous-system events leading to poor digestion. And sadly, I believe it may also be the result of the ongoing presence of antibiotics in the food supply. In the USA alone the Federal Drug Administration (FDA) estimates that the amount of antimicrobial drugs sold and distributed for use in food animals is 29,000,000lbs (13,000,000kg) per year (2008 data) while approximately 7,000,000lbs (3,000,000kg) were sold for human use (2009 data). Sure the rest of the world's consumption is smaller and there are many countries around the world that rigidly (wonderfully) regulate the use of antibiotics in animals, but if animals receive antibiotics, there will be residue in their tissues if we eat them. I believe in the long term, this is then having an effect on the gut bacteria profiles of humans and changing our digestive systems. One of the reasons I believe this is that over the past 14 years, I have observed (OK, so this is not based on scientific research, but it is my observation as a health professional) that almost the only people who don't have gut problems are long-term vegans.

I am not suggesting you all become vegans, unless this resonates for you. I am simply offering you an explanation about why so many women have gut problems today. The combination of stress and the changing gut bacteria profiles is playing a significant role. Please become aware of how much meat you eat, where it comes from, what the animals were fed, and how they were raised, if not for their sake then for yours. Please choose organically reared, pasture-fed meat. The farmers supply what consumers demand. So you can slowly change the world through how you spend your money.

There is now significant scientific evidence that a diet high in plant-based foods not only prevents a significant amount of degenerative disease but can also reverse some of the damage once illnesses such as type 2 diabetes, high blood pressure and heart disease have been diagnosed. Imagine your diet being so powerful.

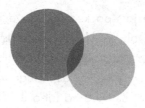

Chapter 9

The Emotional Perspective

Lifting the Veil on
Your Behaviors and Beliefs

So let's now do our best to get to the heart of your matter – to why you feel the need to run your life with urgency. Why you have chosen, and I don't say that lightly, to do what you do and fill your days and nights the way you do. In all honesty, this is my favorite part of what I do because this is where behavioral change is sustained rather than temporary. This is the part that allows you to rest the part of you that is weary and awaken the part of you that is asleep. And optimal health on every level – physical, emotional, and spiritual – is then on offer to you.

Beliefs and behaviors

Every human's greatest fear is that they are not enough and as a result that they won't be loved. We are born this way. It is human psychology 101. Without love a human baby dies. Other animals won't. So this is not some artificial construct that develops over time: it is hardwired into us at our most fundamental level.

Yet, as adults, a life jam-packed with love is delicious but not essential to our survival. So when we live as if love is crucial to our survival, and we do anything and everything we can to avoid being rejected, we live our lives as though we are still children. The trouble is, most of us have no idea that this is what we are doing. We don't realize that the reason we went back to the fridge after a filling dinner last night was to avoid feeling rejected. We've blanketed that with a story that we simply feel like it, or we deserve it having worked so hard all day. But human behavior is the outermost expression of our inner beliefs. It is that simple. Think about that: human behavior is the outermost expression of our inner beliefs, and yet most of us absorbed a set of beliefs before we were even old enough to think for ourselves. And, unless we question these beliefs, they become the default lenses through which we view every situation we ever encounter.

Before our current era of urgency – due to cell phones that we are never without, e-mails requiring a reply within minutes, any food our heart desires at our fingertips, immediate answers to questions via Google, social media posts requiring responses 24/7 – our outermost expressions of not being enough, not being loved, and being rejected, played out in the way we ate, the way we spent money, and the way we spoke to the people around us (to name but a few). In fact, they still do.

Yet, in this age of Google speed, there is now another more obvious, more intense and, in my opinion, potentially even more damaging way that this belief is playing out: women living out the perception that they have to be all things to all people so that they will never, ever be rejected – even though they have no idea that is what they are doing. And to fit everything in, to do all they 'have' to do so that they never, ever let anyone down and risk being 'rejected,' they have gone into overdrive. Otherwise, why would you do it, unless somewhere inside you, you perceived that your life depended on it? Seriously. As I love to say, it's always about love. Everything always is.

Phrases and statements we heard in childhood, such as, 'Don't be so full of yourself; people don't like that' can eventually, if we hear it enough times, become the belief that 'if I want to be loved and accepted, I need to dull and dim and dumb myself down.' Another example might be if we see our parents arguing about money, if money is a source of conflict or never discussed, we give meaning to those situations in the form of beliefs. For example, we might grow up with the belief, 'If I want to be happy in a relationship, I'd better not talk about, not think about, not ever bring up the subject of money.'

We understand situations by giving them meaning. And out of these meanings beliefs are created, which, once formed, become the template for how we see ourselves and how we behave. We then spend the rest of our lives acting as if our subjective beliefs – 'I will never have enough,' 'I must keep the peace,' 'I am lazy/dumb/ unlovable,' 'if I'm not slim/wealthy/a yes girl I won't be loved' – are reality itself. We believe that the way we see our situation is the way things are and that there is no other way. And our actions follow accordingly. Most of us don't even know what we believe. We are so convinced of the rightness of what we see and feel, that we don't realize that we see things as we are, not as they are. It never occurs to us that our belief system is subjective, that there are dozens of ways to interpret the same situation.

To paraphrase Geneen Roth, until we recognize where our beliefs come from, our emotional, financial and spiritual lives will remain frozen in the past, commandeered by beliefs that, for the most part, have no relevance to our current values and the adults we've become.

As much as I love positivity and optimism – I consider myself to have both of those traits – I have not found that it is possible to replace one set of beliefs completely with another by only using what have become known as 'affirmations.' Of course they can help. They can help shift your focus to one of positivity and help you have hope that life can be better. But you can repeat 'I am lovable' a thousand times a day, you can put 'I am super successful' in your car, on your mirror, your computer screen, inside your glasses if you like, but if an earlier belief or conviction of being unlovable is installed in your psyche based on beliefs you created before you could talk, you will only feel better for a moment because you won't actually believe yourself. If you don't do the actual work of deconstructing your fundamental beliefs, the affirmations have no place to land or stick, and their impact is unlikely to be lasting. Please don't get me wrong. By all means do affirmations. They can be nourishment for your soul. I'm simply saying that I have yet to meet someone for whom they alone dismantled what was laid down at the beginning of their time on Earth. Of course be positive and affirm that you are loved. Just explore your beliefs as well for lasting, sustained change.

When people say things like 'Your beliefs determine your experience,' think about this: if you believe that there aren't enough hours in the day or if you believe in being poor or that you will always be fat, that will be your experience. In other words, when you look through 'shattered' lenses, the world looks 'shattered.' It has always been true that we act according to our beliefs and, since the way we act has consequences, our beliefs manifest in the world through various situations. When we act out our beliefs, we see the results of our actions everywhere. It is precisely what happens when you buy a certain colored car of a specific make and model; you suddenly see those cars everywhere! Well guess what? They've always been there. It is simply that now your eyes are primed to notice them. Beliefs work the same way. You see 'evidence' of what you believe everywhere, and you never notice the zillions of examples that make those beliefs null and void.

Clearly it is taking different actions, not just naming beliefs, that leads to change, but in my experience with human health, achieving long-lasting change is impossible without first becoming aware of the deep-seated convictions that are driving your behavior. If you don't realize that the way you are seeing things is not the way they are, if you don't understand that you see yourself, your family, your relationships with food, money, and the world through a version of reality that you developed before you could talk, you believe there is no other way to see and consider the world. You only know what you have experienced and therefore those around you must be hallucinating if they describe it any other way.

Expectations and urgency

I've witnessed the change in people's expectations over the past decade in my practice. Many expect a 90-minute nutrition-focused consultation to 'fix' their entire lives, when they've been using food to cope for at least 15,768,000 minutes (30 years). You have to peel back the layers of the onion through kindness and curiosity about what led you to this point, yet most people believe the only way to sort out their body, for example, is via deprivation and working harder – and if they can't then they will believe that they are a failure before they've even begun.

I've witnessed the massive efforts women make in thousands of clients. They cannot eat any better, even by my exceptionally high nutritional standards.

They cannot move any more than they are already, and their clothes keep getting tighter and tighter. They cannot (until I guide them there) 'see' that there are other ways for bodies to grow or shrink than the calorie equation they have been bombarded with for their entire lives: eat less, move more. My book *Accidentally Overweight* explores precisely this concept: that there is more to fat loss than just calories. If your body gets the message for 16 hours a day, day after day, that your life is in danger and that you must be prepared to run or fight at any moment, your body won't want to use your fat as fuel.

Calming down is the first step for so many women. They need to change the way they eat, exercise, live, think, and behave to ways based on calm. Yet when I explain to them that this panic, this haste, this urgency is what has to change first, many stare at me blankly like I've just asked them to repeat third-grade algebra or recite Latin phrases backward that they've long forgotten. 'What do you mean slowing down will change everything? That means I'll get less done in a day, and you clearly don't understand the pressure I'm under. I run a small country called my life!' 'What do you mean do yoga instead of marathon training – you've got to be crazy – I can't lose weight burning all of the calories I burn doing all of this running... I'll become the size of a house if I only do yoga.' And yet doing the same thing day after day and expecting a different outcome has become known as a definition of insanity. It is time to do things differently and take care of your health in the process.

How to 'do' the slow down

Many women have no idea how to slow down. And when I tell them they actually just have to be, after all we are human beings rather than human doings, I can see from the look on their face that they do their best to hide, that they'd rather go and put their head in a bucket of ice water – that would be easier than surrendering.

So I give them things to do. I offer ways to bring calm and spaciousness back into life. And get them thoroughly exploring, with kindness and curiosity, rather than judgment, what has led them relentlessly to pursue whatever it is that they think they want. You have to do that bit. But then you have to go further. Because it is not about having whatever it is – a larger bank balance, no mortgage, thinner thighs – it is about your perception of how having these things will make you feel. And I am yet to have one single client not pull her veil back and see that, after all, it really is love she is chasing (even though she may or may not already have a life full of love). And in that moment, I always have tears rolling down my face because I know her life will never be the same again. Because in that moment, she has caught a glimpse that what she has been searching for, relentlessly pursuing, is actually within her. And stillness and calm allow you to see it and feel it. She was born that way. She simply forgot. And she will likely forget again, only next time, for not as long. And the strategies help with that. And they make up the final chapter.

So yes, as I said, one definition of insanity is doing the same thing over and over, year after year, and expecting a different outcome. Yet it is like we are in a trance for 10 or 30 years or, for some, a lifetime, doing all we can to make ourselves 'more,' as if we are not enough, yet not seeing that we just keep doing the same thing over and over and our lives never seem to look any different. We think we just require a different diet, or a different exercise program, or less food on our plate, and that will make all the difference. What women need first is to stop dieting.

The science and the psychology behind why diets don't work is a topic that can be a huge source of stress for women – and you can read more about this topic in *Accidentally Overweight*. But at the heart of any form of dieting is usually fear and quite often addiction, whether that is an addiction to food itself or simply an addiction to constantly judging yourself based on the size and shape of your body, regardless of its shape and size. Yet behind all of it is the belief in your own deficiency and the assumption that this can be fixed with an external substance or regime.

People eat unresourcefully for many reasons. It can be a biochemical reason such as low blood glucose that leads someone to polish off too many sweet foods in the middle of the afternoon or after dinner, or it can be emotional, such as when someone creates a meaning of rejection when a colleague gives them constructive feedback at work and they soothe their hurt with food. Or it can be both. Mostly it is both.

So now, knowing how the effect of the rush on the body works, you can truly appreciate why diets don't work, due to both biochemical and emotional factors. Despite the latest fad purporting to be the ultimate weight-loss solution, they simply offer short-term results for a long-term additional gain. Lasting weight loss is never achieved with a fad that starves your body and your soul.

A client recently shared this with me:

> One major thing I've learned since working with you is that I've never really done any self-reflection or looked at why I do the things I do. I thought I was too busy, well, at least, that's the way I perceived it. I thought my answers would be in some pill, website, magazine, or person. It is so easy to direct the focus away from asking yourself hard-hitting questions, but actually only in the short term. When I've looked at myself in the mirror sometimes, I've thought it's as if the lights are on but no one's home. I once had to go to a meeting and they'd phoned the day before to confirm I was coming and to let me know I couldn't park in the car park, yet I still parked in the car park only a day later. It's as if I was hearing words but I'd lost the ability to really listen and process the information.

I was getting appointment dates and times wrong because I'd come to rely on someone texting me to remind me that I have a hair appointment so if they didn't text me, I didn't turn up. It was as if I couldn't remember any details because my mind was fried by all I felt I had to achieve in a day.

• • • • • • • • • • • • • • • • • •

This gorgeous lady took a journey from her head to her heart. It was the shortest distance she ever travelled yet she resisted for some time, denying, unable to see her outward expressions of a cry for love through all she did in her day. She caught a glimpse of it and her life is still full but she is different inside that life.

The to-do list

I'm not saying for one second that there are not things to be done in the day! My goodness, no! I live in the same world as you with a to-do list that is never all crossed off. And I LOVE to cross things off lists. The problem is not the tasks to complete. It is the attitude with which we approach them that influences our health and behind that attitude is a belief.

When you consider your to-do list, instead of approaching it with the attitude of 'oh my goodness, I have to do all of this,' try instead to remember that it is such a privilege that you *get* to do all of this. Many people would be beside themselves to have a life like yours, and this shift in thinking can help you move out of the SNS and into the PNS.

If you have 800 things on your to-do list, you can either approach it with an amped-up, stressed-out, freaking-out-on-the-inside attitude, or you can feel your feet connect to the earth, take a breath in and out that lasts for more than 11 seconds, and acknowledge that you have 800 things on your to-do list. Your headspace, whether it is pent up or calm, does not change what you need to get done in a day. It is what it is. But you can choose your approach.

> **Action**
>
> For calm and centered to become the natural place from which you operate, you need to practice. You need to support yourself with lifestyle choices that promote calm (such as not relying on three double-shot lattes to get you going in the morning) and explore what has led you to live in an anxious state. Is it physical/biochemical, such as too much caffeine before lunch, is it emotional, or is it both?

The good girl

When you curiously open the door on your racing-around state, do you see that you are so scared of getting into trouble because you were raised to be a good girl ('goody two-shoes') that you live your life trying to do everything before anyone even asks you for it? Or before anyone yells at you for not having done it? Or so that no one will criticize you? There is no right or wrong here, no good or bad. This is not a judgment exercise on whether having a goody two-shoes aspect to your personality is a good thing or not. Our behaviors can serve us and also hurt us at the same time.

What I care deeply about is uncovering why you do what you do because then you can choose the behaviors that serve your health and the ones that don't can fall away. Until you explore the destructive behaviors in whatever areas of your life they appear, and get to the heart of them, change will be a battle, and you'll keep returning to your old patterns. Right now my concern is that if you live your life under the cloud of false belief that to never be rejected, you have to be little miss goody two-shoes – and while this will probably make you a kind and likeable person, it also runs the risk of making you a rushing woman, with all of the health consequences that go with that state when you live it long enough. The relentless pursuit of never being rejected – what is it costing you?

Dads and daughters

I'm going to make a big statement. From an emotional standpoint this is the biggest thing I'll say in the whole book. I have yet to meet a rushing woman whose father didn't break her heart. As an adult female, your father is either still your hero or he disappointed you (broke your heart) while you were growing up. You can of course as an adult bring awareness to this area of your life and find peace but my point is, with your father, it is either one way or the other. Hero or heartbreak. If he is still your hero, there won't be room for an intimate male partner to enter your life, or if you are in a relationship, he will play second fiddle to your dad; whatever he does could never compare to what your father would do or what your father would have done. You will also not rush. You will still be your own boss. And you are in the minority of adult women.

On the other hand, if your dad broke your heart that disappointment might have felt as important and painful as death or abuse of any kind toward you or another member of your family or society. Or it may have been that his behavior hurt you but no one else noticed – perhaps with comments that didn't seem hurtful on the surface but could be interpreted that way. Perhaps it was an offhand remark that you 'cost a lot of money' or 'you're just like your mother.' Maybe he was always late to pick you up.

As a child you don't have the emotional maturity to understand that he might be late for a reason – for example working hard to pay for a nice home and a good education, so that you had the best upbringing and opportunities in life. All you know is that he is never there when you want him. And that must be your fault; there must be something unlovable or wrong with you.

> *A close friend of mine felt betrayed by her father and so angry with him for 32 years because he died from cancer when she was nine. As a 41-year-old woman she said to me, 'What kind of father leaves his nine-year-old daughter?' as if he'd simply walked out rather than passed away, making it sound like he had a choice. There she was in front of me as a grown woman speaking the words the nine-year-old felt.*
>
> *When her father died, her mother had to go to work, and my friend saw much less of her and financially their lives were more challenging after he passed away. In my friend's eyes, through her lenses, she believed her dad abandoned her. And she also believed that money was scarce. One of the hardest workers I've ever met, and a woman with a relentless urgency about every aspect of her life, was created from that environment, which when you spell it all out on paper allows you to have great empathy for her. Of course she'd have those personality traits with that kind of past. As an outsider you can completely understand it and have immense compassion for her and how hard it must have been to lose her dad so young.*

· · · · · · · · · · · · · · · · · · ·

You too run behaviors based on your beliefs and I can guarantee you, if you've never looked at this before, you won't have any empathy for yourself. Instead, without realizing it, you will most likely judge yourself and treat yourself with impatience and harshness. Yet it is empathy and kindness toward yourself that you need in order to disarm yourself of the behaviors and beliefs that drive you to say yes to everything, to criticize yourself when you don't live up to the insanely high expectations you set for yourself, the guilt you feel at not calling your mother or your dearest friends enough, not to mention the e-mails you never reply to, and it is also why you've lost the ability to truly and utterly rest... all behaviors that hurt your health.

So when your dad, usually unknowingly, hurt your feelings and you created a belief that for him to love you, you had to be prettier, slimmer, taller, smarter, louder, quieter, more frugal with money, more generous, kinder, sweeter, worry less, care more... whatever you perceived his expectations to be, out of that, much of your behavior has been born.

Remember humans will always do more to avoid pain than to experience pleasure. We are wired that way. We have to be to survive. And that is why when you live your life doing all you can so that your father, whether he is still of this mortal coil or not, will approve, be proud of you and therefore love you, you will be a rushing woman. Technology allows it. You choose it subconsciously, because a part of your nervous system was wired to do so, so that you will survive. Yet an adult, logical mind knows that living so stressfully hurts your health (as I've outlined in previous sections) and can lead to challenging relationships with the people you love the most in this world. So unravel your stories. And see them with new eyes. It is time to see the world as it really is, not through the eyes of your child self. It is time to take responsibility for yourself and your choices and understanding what drives those choices (avoiding rejection) changes everything.

Reflect

As you begin to explore your stories (as opposed to reality), talk to yourself the way you would speak to a precious child, for with such tenderness, the fear of not being enough dissolves and is no longer the driving force of your behavior in that moment. And the more consciously you live, the more you are present in each moment, you will so clearly see that you are wonderful.

There is not a little girl in the world who is not born knowing that she is wonderful. Not in a conceited way, just a precious kind of way. And we lose that. It is part of the human condition. Girls lose it at different times, but we all lose that knowing. And I believe we spend the rest of our lives trying to feel like that again, using food, shopping, achievement at work, or achievement at keeping people happy to do so. Yet if you knew who you truly are, you would be in awe of yourself.

None of this means that the mother-daughter relationship doesn't affect us, as the same set-up in our nervous system can unconsciously occur when we are growing up. But I've just seen it far more often in the father-daughter relationship over the past 20 years of working with women. As the novelist Allison Pearson accurately describes the 'dad thing' in *I Don't Know How She Does It*, so many of us are 'pursuing the elusive ghost of paternal love.'

And it's important that you know that none of these schisms need to come from trauma or tragedy. You can grow up in a calm and peaceful home and you will still create a meaning that you have to do something to be loved (rather than just be, as very young children do). It happens to everyone. In fact, it happens for everyone. And the reason it is a gift, that we get the opportunity to explore and alter in adulthood, is because no one would ever contribute anything if they truly lived every moment perceiving they are unconditionally loved.

Who is affected by Rushing Woman's Syndrome?

When the enormity of the health consequences that arise from the perception of pressure and the need for urgency hit me, I first questioned where does it come from, what drives it, and who does it affect? I've outlined my take on these three questions above but as an addition to the third query I offer you this.

Initially when I reflected on the demographic affected by RWS I thought it was Western women in their thirties and forties but on observing patients with this in mind for the past five years, I can now very clearly see that most women are not immune to it. I've met women in their late sixties, some of the kindest, most caring, gracious women I have ever met in fact, who go into a panic on the inside as soon as anyone asks them to do anything.

One woman in particular springs to mind and she is evidence that RWS is not just the result of the rapid increase in the technology available to us, as many of the women I work with are not constantly using technology.

One of my female clients, who didn't use e-mail and only used her cell phone to keep in touch with relatives overseas, saw me for severe diarrhea that was very debilitating. When she went for a walk in the mornings, she couldn't make it to the end of the street without having to run back home and use the lavatory with an intense urgency. After tests with a gastroenterologist revealed nothing amiss with her bowels, I asked her about the relationships she shared with the people closest to her. She said her children were lovely (both were adults and lived overseas) but she merely tolerated her husband, as he was a tyrant. He'd had multiple affairs that she knew about, and raised his voice and overreacted at the slightest mishap. She appeared happy on the outside and yet on the inside she was wired and she did everything in her life with immense haste.

She felt like she loved him, she said. But the reality was that she lived in fear of him – not physical abuse but emotional. She said she chose to stay because she couldn't bear the thought of losing the home she had created over the past

40 years. When I asked her if she felt like he loved her she said no and he hadn't for 37 years and she'd done everything possible with her appearance, her body, her cooking, and her immense level of care in an attempt to earn his love. And the desire for his love spills over into the need to keep everyone happy – to keep the peace.

• • • • • • • • • • • • • • • • • • •

And this lovely lady's story illustrates perfectly where all the urgency, the rushing, and the intensity with which we as women approach our to-do list, comes from. Earning love. Never being rejected. Oh and too much caffeine. But I've barked on about that enough already.

I express no judgment here. I simply want to demonstrate that rushing has become the way so many women run their days, and it is not just the result of technology and the immediacy that it often 'requires' of us. Technology has simply made it easier for people like me (health professionals) to see it. If you try to fill something that can't be filled with what you are using, the emptiness never goes away and you keep wanting more. Only you usually don't see this until you explore your inner world.

Beliefs and thoughts lead to feelings and feelings lead to actions. Feelings can also lead to beliefs, which then lead to actions. We respond to other people, treat our children, mates, strangers, coworkers, and people on the street based on our beliefs. Everything we do, every word that we utter, every relationship we have is an expression of what we believe.

A lady, Sonia, who worked with me part-time recently told me she wished she could work with me full-time and forever. I smiled with her and asked her why, and she replied because I am always happy, I talk to her kindly, and I laugh with her. I asked her what it is like at her other jobs and she said they hardly ever smile and mostly don't speak to her unless they have to give her instructions. And it made me wonder where courtesy and kindness are disappearing to in this world. And it led me to write this on Facebook:

> There is a story behind every person. There is a reason why they are the way they are. Do your best to consider this always, as it helps us to not judge others. The Dalai Lama said it beautifully: 'The basic foundation of humanity is compassion and love. This is why, if even a few individuals simply try to create mental peace and happiness within themselves and act responsibly and kind-heartedly towards others, they will have a positive influence in their community.'

* * * * * * * * * * * * * * * * * * *

'The more you recognize the best in others, the more gratitude you have for the gifts that make them precisely who they are. The more you express that gratitude, the more alive and fulfilled you feel – and the more you're able to appreciate the best in yourself.'

TONY ROBBINS

Not enough

The belief that you are not, and don't have, enough might manifest in unkind behavior toward people you actually love. It may manifest as a desperate feeling for more... more of anything or anyone... which might show up in your life as eating too much, spending beyond your means or frequent, brief intimate encounters. A belief that you don't have enough will make you utterly blind to, and entirely callous about, those who have less, because you believe that you are one of them. When you are caught in a trance of deficiency, your task, your only task, is to do whatever it takes to get more. If fortune throws a significant amount of money in your lap you won't see it. You will find a way to make it disappear so that the world you live in will be congruent with your beliefs.

With decades of experiments examining everything from the efficacy of wrinkle creams to observations of car colors, scientists have discovered that we don't believe what we see, rather we see what we believe. Again, we don't believe what we see... we see what we believe. Until you are willing to name your beliefs, either because circumstances force your hand or because you wake up to the pain of seeing through shattered lenses or because you are sick of living your life in a great big rush and the subsequent health consequences, you will continue to act on your self-created version of reality, which is why women who believe that all men cheat will see 'evidence' of it in the way he interacts with every female he comes into contact with, even though he adores her. It is why lottery winners tend to blow through their cash and end up broke... even with millions they believe they are poor, and actions always conform to beliefs.

Unless you name your beliefs you will continue to believe that your version of reality is the way that it is, not the way you choose it to be based on your beliefs. Naming beliefs and exploring the feelings that arise is an ongoing, exciting, heart-opening process.

Awaken the part of you that is asleep

There are times when rushing serves a brilliant purpose and when it is short-lived, there is no problem for our physical and emotional health. We cope without a hitch. But when you live in that state day after day, year after year, it can take an immense toll on your health.

With so many of the women I see in my practice and at my weekends and events, I can see that the rush is at the heart of the health problems they've come to see me about. Although they firstly either deny they are stressed, despite their blood tests showing they are, and tell me this is just how their life is, or they agree to slow down ('funny you say that, my mother always tells me to slow down,' they'll say) but they don't. Nothing about their lifestyle changes. And the best diet in the world, the best supplements, or the best exercise plan, won't even touch the sides when your sympathetic nervous system is always dominant. And to allow your parasympathetic nervous system, the rest-and-digest arm, to do its vital work, you first need to understand what SNS dominance is actually doing to you and therefore why you need to change and then, secondly, you need to explore the emotional landscape of why you feel the need to do everything with urgency.

As you now understand from the previous chapters in this book, we have very ancient hormonal mechanisms in action inside our bodies that believe they know better than you when it comes to your survival. Your body can be your biggest teacher if you learn how to decipher the messages it is communicating to you. And your behaviors, extra body fat or an unjustified panicked perception of life, are sometimes simply vehicles of communication, doing their best to remind you to rest the part of you that is weary and awaken the part of you that is asleep. And mostly the part of women that has gone to sleep is our belief, our deep knowing of how precious we are and that we deserve nothing but the best care, the utmost kindness and nurturing, and nourishment for our body, mind, and soul; gifts we can choose to give ourselves every single day.

And for the mothers in particular, the women for whom guilt has become a way of life, I ask you to remember this sentiment... you are the best mother your child will ever have. You are their barometer and their compass in this world. And every single child thinks that their mother is absolutely wonderful.

Reflect

As you explore your beliefs about who you have to be to be loved and who you can never be, you'll see part of why you have your personality and make some of the choices you do. Why do you do what you do, even though you know what you know? Usually it is to avoid emotional pain. Bring awareness to this. Bring compassion to yourself. Bring curiosity instead of judgment and instead wonder what might have led you to make a particular choice. Curiosity opens us to insight. Judgment shuts it down. Get back in touch with what you were born knowing: that you are precious, and treat yourself accordingly.

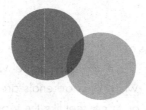

Chapter 10
Counting the Cost
*The Impact of Rush
on Your Wellbeing*

It is with even more love and respect for women everywhere that I write this chapter. I believe many women are unaware of what living as a rushing woman is doing to them on a physical level – PMS, debilitating menopause, IBS, poor sleep, 'unexplained' weight gain – as well as on an emotional level – feeling anxious, mood swings, anger, impatience, and easily laying blame for things on other people. And it is all of this that can easily lead a woman to dislike herself, judge herself, and hold a tension in her body that is destructive to her health and her relationships... not fun and lighthearted stuff which is partly why I opened this chapter with a gentle statement. We women are truly amazing. And we can do anything. My concern is that for so many women, their perceived need to be all things to all people is taking its toll in a much bigger way than most may realize.

PMS

The link between stress and PMS is undeniable from both a scientific perspective and also from my experience with clients. And as you now understand, when your adrenals are churning out stress hormones, your body does not feel like the world is a 'safe' place, so you may find it harder to bring a baby into your stressful world, if your adrenal production of progesterone is compromised. Of course pregnancy can still occur when you are stressed as our emotional and primal drive to reproduce is also very powerful. However, with the amping-up effects of adrenalin combined with the loss of the antianxiety agent progesterone, you have a biochemical recipe to rush and the basis of PMS and some cases of 'unexplained infertility'.

As I outlined in Chapter 5, the other biochemical picture that leads to PMS is estrogen being dominant to progesterone, not necessarily due to poor adrenal production of progesterone but through excess estrogen. Once estrogen has done its job in your body over a month, the liver decides whether to excrete the estrogen or recycle it. Recycling is far more likely when the liver has to prioritize the detoxification and excretion of substances that the body perceives as far more toxic to our health than estrogen. The body doesn't see estrogen as a poison because your own ovaries and fat cells make it. However, due to our environmental exposure to estrogens and estrogen-like substances, such as those in plastics and pesticides, not to mention synthetic versions of estrogen found in the oral contraceptive pill (OCP) and hormone replacement therapy (HRT), we are being exposed to more estrogen than ever before in human history. Combine that with women's increased intake of some of the major 'liver loaders,' which include alcohol, caffeine, and some refined sugars, such as sucrose and high fructose corn syrup and any of its derivatives, and you have an additional recipe for the rush and another form of PMS due to a congested liver.

Anger

I do not believe that any emotion is bad. The way we express emotions can, however, be constructive or destructive; serve the world or not. Combine the feelings of impatience, frustration, and anger welling up inside a woman who perceives there are not enough hours in the day to do all she needs to do – which subconsciously she believes she has to do so that she will keep everyone happy and that her life depends on this – with a congested liver, a whole pile of stress hormones, often with negligible progesterone, and while we are at it, let's throw a couple of adrenalin-inducing coffees in and a dusty head from too much alcohol the night before, and you have a woman on the verge of becoming a cyclone at any conceivable moment. And when she lets fly, it will most likely be over something that in the big scheme of things doesn't really matter – like the butter being left out or a wet towel on the bathroom floor. And who is most likely to be on the receiving end of her explosion? The people she loves the most in this world: her family, her roommates, or her colleagues. Mostly, it is family. And as the beautiful Buddhist saying goes: 'You will not be punished for your anger; you will be punished by your anger.'

If the description above rings true for you, if you scream at your children or your beloved and wish you didn't, and if this is harder to control in the lead-up to your period, please understand that the cocktail of hormones described above is powerful and likely to be behind your PMS-based anger.

You'll find more reasons why alcohol is part of the picture in Rushing Woman's Syndrome below but if you suffer with PMS and you drink wine, stop. Stop for three months. Your liver is screaming at you to change your ways. This is even more important if your breasts form lumps easily and if this is worse premenstrually. If taking a break from alcohol feels impossible to you, double-check that this is the case. It is, after all, only a drink, and three months is a tiny amount of time in your long life. If you still say it is impossible for you, then switch to gin or vodka with soda, and add fresh lemon or lime. Measure the nip of spirits and limit it to two per day making sure you have a minimum of two alcohol-free days every week. Also apply the strategies for estrogen dominance outlined in Chapter 5.

Finally, please understand that you need to make some changes, not only for yourself and your physical health, but also for the sake of those you love. They don't understand what is behind your outbursts. They think it is about them and that they have to change who they are for you to love them. Our children need us to take responsibility for our behaviors and, as you now understand, your behaviors are simply the outermost expression of your beliefs.

Reflect

Be honest with how you express your emotions and who is feeling the brunt of any PMS-induced rage. This is not an exercise in self-guilt or self-reflection; it is simply about awareness and making a commitment to take action to resolve any ongoing issues.

The following is an e-mail written to me by a patient, who I will call Elise, who came to see me for help with her PMS. She said it was so bad that, even though she had a lovely husband, she wanted to divorce him for two weeks out of every month. She was prepared to do whatever I asked her, she told me, if it would help her be relieved of her PMS, yet when I asked her to take a break from alcohol for two menstrual cycles, she resisted. However, to her credit she did it and this is part of the e-mail she wrote to me at the end of what turned out to be three very insightful months. I have Elise's permission to reproduce this part of her note.

When you asked me to take a break from alcohol for two months I felt like crying. Instead I did what I always do, as you pointed out, which was to get angry. Three months have now passed and I cannot tell you how different I feel. I never really dreamt that I would be free of PMS. But it is gone. The thing is, part of me is devastated at what I used to be like. Thank goodness for my husband because he keeps reminding me that the way I used to behave can all be in the past now. But I'm horrified at what I used to be like. And I couldn't even see it. But now I see it in other women. Some of them are my friends. They scream at their kids at a level that is not OK. Children don't understand that there is a substance that changes your personality. They just know you are you and that you are their whole world and that sometimes you seem different and to a child that means that they must have done something wrong. I don't want women to think I'm judging them because it is as if they can't help it, let alone see it. At the same time, though, I think they are behaving like a child themselves for not taking responsibility for their actions. If alcohol is what is behind someone yelling at or ignoring their children then they need to stop drinking.

· · · · · · · · · · · · · · · · · · ·

The importance of patience and kindness

The Dalai Lama offers brilliant insights about anger. He says it is a blind energy that (momentarily) destroys the part of your brain that is able to judge right or wrong. He says anger can't see reality. He says that to face a problem, we must know reality and the mind needs to be calm to investigate reality. Otherwise we can't see objectively. To use human intelligence properly, the mind needs to be calm. Anger destroys inner peace and the ability to investigate reality. And Elise's road to have the 'blindness' reversed was dietary change, a significant part of which was not consuming alcohol for a period of time.

A raised voice, regardless of its intention, signals to a human nervous system that there is danger. If we yell at a child to warn them of danger, they get the message. If a child is yelled at because they dropped a glass by accident and then the next day they are on the receiving end of another raised voice because they forgot to take their water bottle to school and then two days later they are again yelled at for not dressing themselves warmly enough, a pattern starts to emerge in their life, and they form beliefs about who they are, about what kind of person they must be to be on the receiving end of harshness from someone who is always right: their parent.

Please, please, please know this is not designed to elicit guilt. It is designed to wake you up if this is part of you that has gone to sleep or is blinded by your anger. Please move beyond guilt if that is where you have gone in your head and hear my point. My point is that it is incredibly hard to express kindness when you feel broken. It is very difficult to practice patience when you are under immense time pressures. Yet patience and kindness are crucial here.

Alcohol

I meet women who truly believe that there is nothing harmful in drinking 12 bottles of wine a week. There is not a woman on the planet whose body, mind, or soul can handle that much alcohol, week after week. Most women I meet overdrink — that is they consume amounts of alcohol deemed by scientific research to be unsafe. Unsafe in relation to what? Most notably cancer. Scientific research has unquestionably linked the regular overconsumption of alcohol to six major cancers: breast, colon, stomach, liver, throat, and esophageal.[1-3] It worries me enormously the way so many women, both of childbearing age and those who are postmenopausal, regularly overconsume alcohol. Please wake up and make a change in this area before a health crisis demands that you do. You don't need this book or a health professional to tell you that you drink too much if you do. You know better than anyone else. So now please let your own intuition drive you to make a behavioral change.

How do you do this? You pick an avenue to start. For example, you might choose to begin with the way you eat. Many people drink as soon as they get home because they are hungry and thirsty. Have a glass of water and a handful of nuts instead and see if you still want the wine. Or significantly amp up the green plant food content of what you eat each day, as the bitter taste base of green vegetables helps taste buds desire less alcohol (and often less sugar). Check out my cookbooks *Real Food Chef, Real Food Kitchen* and *Sweet Food Story* for more information about this and practical recipes to support you.

Alternatively you could simply decide to take a break from drinking alcohol for one month. Or two. Or three. I've had women who initially felt like this would be impossible, do this without blinking an eye. And feel so proud of themselves for doing so. And then if you choose to bring alcohol back, drink only one or two days a week and not every week. Or save it for super special occasions.

Alternatively approach overdrinking from an emotional perspective. Ask yourself to finish the sentence 'Alcohol is...' or 'wine is...' and keep going until you feel a little shiver down your spine or get goose bumps (goose pimples), which signal that you have hit on your truth. And you will see that you have constructed a story about what this drink is to you. So then ask yourself what the other ways you could feel this way are. And bring more of that into your life. Or simply see that you subconsciously created a story about alcohol and why you 'need' it, to get you through a tough time. It's just that you kept using it this way and now it is the only way you know how to, for example, relax. You have not always relied on alcohol to relax. There are plenty of other ways. Besides, when you rush less, which you will once you have gotten to the heart of your matter (see Chapter 9, page 157) you will feel far less amped up and stressed and you will 'need' alcohol to relax far less often. In fact, you will look at your life differently, through a different set of lenses, and see that a relaxed state of mind is available to you at every given moment.

Here are some more facts about alcohol. I simply share these with you so that you understand the way it impacts us from the inside out. When you are better informed, it helps you to make choices for yourself from a place of self-care, rather than feeling like some bossy boots nutritional biochemist told you to do so. When we make changes that well up from inside us from a place of self-care, changes are most likely to be sustained, enjoyed and embraced.

Alcohol can lead to:

- Increased body fat

- Cellulite

- Less energy and vitality

- Worse bouts of PMS

- Mood fluctuations

- Lack of mental clarity

- Feeling like you can't cope – you don't feel hungover but your ability to deal with what comes your way each day leaves you frustrated, irritated or sad

January might see some making big statements about their health and alcohol reduction or avoidance. Some prefer February to take a break, as they've worked out it has the fewest number of days! Rascals! I know others who do Dry July or Oct-sober in October.

People drink for wide and varied reasons. For some, it is the way they socialize, or the way they wind down from the day. Some use alcohol to distract themselves from thoughts and feelings they'd rather avoid. It can be a way that people cope. Regardless of the reason, many people overconsume alcohol without even realizing it.

A standard drink in many Western countries is 10g (0.35oz) of alcohol, however that comes – a 330ml bottle of 4 percent beer, a 30ml nip of spirits, 170ml of champagne, and it is a measly 100ml of wine – about four swallows! Next time you pour yourself a glass of wine, measure it, and see what your natural pour is. For most, it is considerably more than a measure and, as a result, many people are overdrinking without even realizing.

We have long heard the heart-health benefits of red wine publicly sung, and many justify their drinking behaviors based on this. 'I'm looking after my heart' they'll say. Current recommendations from heart organizations suggest no more than two standard drinks per day with two alcohol-free per week is OK for women, and three standard drinks per day and two AFDs is acceptable for men. And cancer-based organizations from around the world, which base their advice on evidence-based scientific studies, typically 'recommend' even less is consumed: two drinks maximum for men and one drink maximum for women per day, with a minimum of two AFDs per week.[1-3]

I'm not suggesting you don't drink alcohol if you currently do, although many people benefit from reducing it or omitting it – particularly women with an excess of estrogen or a family history of cancer, particularly breast cancer. This is due to the undeniable link between the consistent overconsumption of alcohol and breast cancer. Research has shown this time and time again, and for many years now. Yet we rarely hear about it. The American Cancer Society suggests that even a few drinks per week may increase a person's risk (of breast cancer).[21]

Of course alcohol consumption can be immensely pleasurable for those who partake. I simply want to appeal to you to get honest with yourself about how alcohol affects you. You know in your heart if you drink too much and when it is negatively impacting your health. Where you want to bring curiosity – not judgment – is to why you consider treating yourself with a lack of care when you know you are consistently doing something that hurts you.

Alcohol can also affect the way we relate to those we love the most in the world, and of course it affects how you feel about yourself. So, if you drink, consume your beverage of choice mindfully and certainly enjoy it, rather than for the misconstrued message that alcohol is good for your health.

The human body cannot excrete alcohol; it has to be converted into acetaldehyde by the liver, and then the acetaldehyde can be excreted. This is the lousy substance that gives us a headache the day after too much the night before. If the liver doesn't do its job properly and alcohol accumulates in the blood, we can go into a coma and die. Alcohol is that poisonous. And I don't say that lightly. But, thankfully, the liver jumps to action and starts the conversion process and we can carry on. Over time, though, this can take its toll.

If people drink daily (or, for some, even just regularly), the liver can be so busy dealing with alcohol – a priority substance to be excreted – that other substances the liver has to change don't get the attention they need and are instead recycled. Estrogen and cholesterol are two examples. It is often the recycling of these substances that leads to their elevated levels in the body, which can lead to health challenges.

If you want to cut back or cut out alcohol for a while, or even if you just want to break your habit of regular drinking, you might like to still pour yourself a drink at the time you would typically imbibe, and do what you would normally do. Sit and chat to your partner, make dinner, talk on the phone to a friend. So often we have mentally linked the glass of wine to a pleasurable activity (or as a way to 'cope' with the 'witching hour') when it is actually the pleasurable activity that we don't want to miss out on! So have sparkling water in a wine glass, with some fresh lime or lemon if that appeals, and add a few more alcohol-free days to your life.

Please get honest with yourself about how alcohol affects you and those around you. And with kindness toward yourself, always kindness, take steps to drink much less than you do now, if this has rung true for you. From a calorie perspective, one glass of wine is the equivalent of three slices of bread. And I've met countless women who tell me that they couldn't possibly eat a slice of even good-quality bread in their day, yet they will drink half to a full bottle of wine (or more) many nights of the week.

This is part of a vicious cycle because when you wake with a dusty head, you reach for coffee to clear the dust, another liver loader and adrenalin-production enhancer. Change these two dietary behaviors alone, and you will naturally rush a whole lot less and enjoy the health benefits that come with less urgency in your life.

Please, please get your health, starting with the liver loaders, on track so that you can give your mind every opportunity to be calm. I believe that is our duty, that this is part of our responsibility to ourselves, to others, including our children. And that is how you change the world.

Here's how to recognize that the liver needs support.

- Liver roll – an increased roll of fat high up under the bra of women, under the sternum of men

- Tender point in the center of your torso (this can also indicate gallbladder issues and I've observed that it can occur after heartbreak or massive disappointment. If your gallbladder has been removed, you now have no place to store bile so your liver has to make bile on demand. As you now understand, the liver already has a lot to do, so this situation often benefits from additional liver support)

- Short temper; easily irritated

- Episodes or feelings of intense anger

- 'Liverish,' gritty, impatient behavior

- PMS

- Cellulite (lymphatic or cortisol-related also)

- Overheating easily

- Floaters in your vision (may also be related to iron deficiency)

- Waking around 2 a.m.

- Sleep that is worse on an evening you consume alcohol

- Waking up feeling hot in the night

- Not hungry for breakfast when you first get up in the morning

- Prefer to start your day with coffee

- Elevated cholesterol

- Estrogen-dominant symptoms in the second half of your menstrual cycle

- You bloat easily

- Drinking alcohol daily

- Daily long-term caffeine consumption

Irritable bowel syndrome (IBS)

Irritable bowel syndrome or any other digestive system disorder can make being intimate with the person you love the least appealing thing on the planet. And without going into enormous details here, most husbands link physical intimacy to you loving them. And sure they might understand for a couple of days that you aren't in the mood, but when those few days stretch into him perceiving that you haven't felt like being physically intimate with him for months or years, that can be tough on a relationship. Not to mention that you can also miss out on the closeness and pleasure.

I know many women who have searched for years to solve their battle with a bloated or unpredictable tummy. So please know ladies, there is a reason. And as I outlined earlier, the most common ones are SNS dominance, a parasite infection/gut dysbiosis, or food intolerance or two or three of these factors. So apply the suggested strategies and have your tummy no longer be a source of your discomfort and interior panic.

Reflect

If your digestive system problems are the way your stress and your SNS dominance play out, explore whether this is having an impact on your wider life. What does it mean for you socially? At work? Are you always on edge making sure there is a toilet nearby? Do you decline special invitations so you don't have to risk having an upset tummy and so miss seeing people who uplift you?

Debilitating menopause

If you have been in SNS dominance for many years and your sex hormone production starts to change, menopause is far more likely to be challenging and potentially debilitating for you, with some of the major symptoms being hot flashes, interrupted sleep, and vaginal dryness.

Given the focus on what being a rushing woman is costing you, I simply want to encourage you to see that it is crucial to sort out the RWS drivers before going into menopause so you are more likely to experience more subtle changes in your health parameters and the way you feel. Going into menopause with SNS dominance sets you up to have poor adrenal production of progesterone, the hormone with significant antianxiety and antidepressant properties. Once menopause arrives, ovarian production of hormones ceases and in an ideal world, you would go from having good progesterone production to a small amount from your adrenal glands. Instead, what I see every day of my working life, are women who go from having a progesterone reading of <0.5 (so virtually zero progesterone on a day of their cycle when ideally there would be 25 units of progesterone) to the same super low reading in menopause. Without good adrenal production of progesterone you have nothing to fall back on when ovarian production ceases. So sort out the rush before menopause begins.

If you are currently passing through perimenopause or menopause, and you went into it with all of the classic signs of RWS, there is still so much you can do to support your health (see Chapter 11, page 199). And if you are now postmenopausal and still feel panicky on the inside, again the strategies outlined in Chapter 11 will serve you.

> **Action**
>
> There is so much you can do to support your health. See your body as a barometer. It does not have a voice but it will always give you symptoms to let you know if it is unhappy and wants you to pay attention to something. And often it is to your very own intuition.

Poor sleep

What is living in SNS dominance costing you? It is often the quality of your sleep. And when our sleep quality is compromised, so many aspects of our health are impacted too. When you awake in the morning not feeling refreshed and alert, you tend to make poorer food choices; most often you will reach for the high-sugar foods and/or caffeinated drinks believing you need them in order to keep going. So poor sleep can affect your desire to take good care of yourself.

When you don't sleep well, long-term, all of your pituitary hormones can also be affected, which as you now know can affect every cell of your body (see Chapter 7, page 120). Thyroid hormones, sex hormones, and of course stress hormones have been found to be higher in those who don't sleep well. The flipside is that adrenalin, one of your stress hormones, does not want you to sleep, as it is communicating to every cell of your body that your life is in danger so the last thing it believes is that it is safe for you to sleep deeply.

When clients come to me for help with their sleep, the majority of women are SNS dominant and until we can alter that, the deep, restful, restorative sleep does not return on a regular basis. You need to do all you can to allow your body to feel 'safe.' And sleep will come.

Poor sleep also has a relationship with your other stress hormone, cortisol. As was outlined in Chapter 4 (see page 48), cortisol levels naturally fall away in the evening and allow you to fall asleep. Cortisol naturally starts to rise around 2 a.m., and sleep is less likely to be as deep after this time. Going to bed by 10:30 p.m., at the latest, is ideal for restorative sleep. But what rushing woman is going to do that?

E-mails

I'll say it again – when you tell me that you delete e-mails off your phone while in the bathroom because that's good time management, I can tell you, with love and respect, that you are a rushing woman. E-mails can infiltrate every corner of your life if you allow them.

I was recently able to witness New Zealand women's Internet habits when I announced that I was holding a second cooking school (the first one sold out two hours prior to this one being announced). The announcement went out via e-mail at around 4:50 p.m. and with a limited number of seats, I had to watch the sales carefully. The initial influx of sales happened up until around 6 p.m. My guess was that women then either drove home from work or began preparing dinner. There were very few sales 7–8:30 p.m. and then, within the next hour, the event was all sold out.

And it made me think – where once, after dinner, women connected with the people they love, did household tasks, read or relaxed, they now finish their evening duties and head to their computer to do e-mails, use social media, or do more work that they brought home from the office. Where once, weekends were for recreation, connection, shopping, gardening, and perhaps solitude and time for reflection, now the work, the e-mails, and the social media use continue. Or if it doesn't continue, it is often on a woman's mind so that by the time she gets to Sunday, if she hasn't done any of these things over the weekend, women will tell me that a mild panic sets in with the anticipation of what will be in their inbox the next day. No nervous system on the planet can handle panic long-term.

Sure there are times when e-mails and social media are great fun and bring us pleasure. But when they compromise your health because you dread the sheer number or what they will contain, there is a bigger thing at play, and the emotions section of this book is crucial for you (see Chapter 9, page 157). Too much time spent on your computer can cost you precious moments with the people you love the most in this world. It's just that we forget to notice this along the way.

Body fat

A rushing woman may be slim, skinny, or overweight. In *Accidentally Overweight* the focus was on the nine factors that determine whether humans use body fat as their fuel effectively or not. So to capture a part of the essence of that message that is particularly relevant to RWS, I offer you this:

It is as if many women's bodies never feel 'safe' enough to use fat as fuel for they are constantly on red alert, ready to act the split second the next 'crisis' happens. Humans burn fat effectively when we have what I call a balanced nervous system and, as you now know, that is when we can switch appropriately between being SNS dominant and PNS dominant and also sit comfortably and happily in what is known as homeostasis... when your body is in balance. Create the 'safety,' re-establish optimal health, and the body fat-burning will naturally and effortlessly follow.

Here's what I know...

This was the hardest chapter to write because I know some of this information may have been hard for some of you to read. I intend no offense, no judgment, no guilty responses, only insights and experiences from my work and my amazing clients. I want you to be happy and I want you to experience amazing health. I want you to truly know, feel, and experience the incredible woman that you are. It is time to treat yourself with the care you deserve.

The following is a gorgeous piece called *Here's What I Know*, written by the talented Kate Northrup, a woman with a deep care for other women that I met at a conference in the USA recently. She wrote this on a piece of paper and found it in her car when she cleaned it not so long ago. Her sentiments echo many of my own. I encourage you to be inspired by her words and to create your own 'Here's what I know...'

- Doing something for the money never ends up being worth it.

- If it's not a hell yes, it's a no.

- You are valuable because you exist. Period. (Or, full stop if you're British).

- You are enough. You always have been. You always will be.

- Your place of greatest ease and joy will also be your place of greatest service.

- It's OK to sleep for 10 hours or more a night from time to time. In fact, it's critical.

- No accomplishment or moment of recognition will ever replace feeling loved, by yourself or anyone else.

- You know. You always know.

- The fact that it feels good is reason enough to move every day. The fact it will tone your ass and make your waist smaller are mere side effects.

- Organizing your life around what feels good is the single wisest choice you can make.

- Saying yes to someone simply because you don't want to disappoint them is not only unfair to you, it's unfair to them.

- Sleep, water, movement, greens, and a good cry cure almost anything.

- Anything worth taking seriously is worth making fun of. (Thanks, Mom.)

- Paying attention to your money is a profound act of self-love.

- It turns out that life is happening right now.

- Loving yourself more is the best place to start to solve any problem.

- You can't judge and have an open heart at the same time.

- Nothing is random. Everything happens for a reason.

- Your body is wise beyond what you could possibly imagine. Listen to her. She will lead you home every time.

- Home is not a place.

Your turn!

What do you know?

What can you count on no matter what?

Reflect

Reflect on what some of your choices are costing you, or those you love. Does the rush primarily affect your physical wellbeing – your quality of sleep, your energy, digestion or how your clothes fit? Or does the rush impact you emotionally far more powerfully or detrimentally? Are you intense or aggressive or overreact with the people you love the most in this world, or with strangers? Or do you tend to withdraw in overwhelm as a result of the rush? Bring curiosity (not judgment) to how the rush is affecting the many aspects of your life.

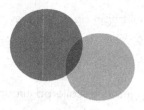

Chapter 11

From Rush to Calm

Solutions

I t is always tempting when reading a book like this to jump straight to the solutions, especially for a rushing woman! When you think that you don't have the time to read the whole book, you just want to cut to the chase and get the answers, then put answers into action and get your results. Right? Umm, well hear me out.

First, if you've come to this chapter first, I cannot encourage you enough to return to the beginning of this book and read it from cover to cover. Science teaches us that you first have to know why you need to change something because when the why is strong enough, the change is a natural follow-through. If the solutions offered here were simply a list of instructions, then this section will only be additions to your never-ending to-do list that you may (or not) do for two weeks or two months, but before long you will return to your old ways and the health consequences that potentially go with them. Without knowing why I might be asking you to focus on your breathing every day for the next six weeks, you might do this for a brief period but as soon as you get beyond busy, you will feel like you don't have time and the breathing sessions will cease and the rush will begin again... if it ever stopped in the first place. So to that end, you need to know why I am making the following suggestions.

Second, there are suggestions scattered through each chapter that won't necessarily be repeated here.

Third, I believe that you are more likely to take action to care for yourself when a particular section of this book speaks directly to you. When that happens, when you feel like I've read your diary or your mind, or like I've caught a glimpse of your life, or perhaps you got goose bumps, laughed, or cried, then you are far more compelled to act, than if you simply read my recommendations below.

I begin with a set of general suggestions designed to help your biochemistry switch from rushing to calm. These will support all of the body systems discussed as part of the rush. And I remind you to please spend some time in solitude, with a journal by your side if that appeals, exploring what may have bubbled to the surface for you while reading the chapter on emotions, in particular (see Chapter 9, page 157). Once you catch a glimpse of where the rush originated, the immense power to change your whole life is in your hands, and change naturally flows from this space.

Small changes can have powerful results. Imagine that your life's destiny was going to run like a set of railway tracks, with the left track remaining a consistent width apart from the right track. Let's say these imaginary tracks are set to run from New York to Dallas. From the point you begin to make lifestyle changes, even if you only change what you do or how you think by two degrees, the left and right tracks will start to veer away from each other. At first they are just a few steps apart but after a few months they are miles apart and after a year, you are worlds apart from where you would have been had you not initiated change. The right track, the path of your previous destiny, will still arrive in Dallas but by adopting your changes and sustaining them, the left track will now arrive in Miami. Worlds apart.

Restorative foundations: Eating, movement, sleep, and action

Eating the right foods, including some yin movement, getting restorative sleep, and taking small daily actions are the vital foundations for switching your body from rush to rest.

Restorative eating

It is very difficult to be kind, compassionate, and patient with others when you fill yourself with stimulants and foods that contain very little nutritional value. I believe that if each of us embraces compassion, kindness, and patience, there will be no need for violence in any form. But if humans fill themselves with too much caffeine, alcohol, and 'dead' food, it makes it much harder for them biochemically to access these gentle emotional states consistently. A real food diet allows you to explore your emotional landscape with clarity and free yourself from patterns that no longer serve you. Food becomes part of you and the nutrients from food drive every chemical reaction inside of you.

Choose whole, real foods that nourish you and watch your physical, as well as your emotional, health shine.

Eat real food the way it comes in nature as often as you can

- Remember nature gets it right whereas human intervention can get it wrong so avoid processed food, artificial colors, sweeteners, flavorings and preservatives.

- When you are in control of your food (i.e. it is up to you to choose), you 'zig' and eat nourishing food; when you are at someone else's house for dinner (for example) you eat what they serve and you 'zag' so that you still get to socialize without compromising your health.

- Let's say you eat 35 times per week: three main meals and two snacks, seven days per week. (Some of you will eat more or less frequently than that.) If, at the moment, seven out of your 35 eating occasions are made from whole, real foods, if you just include one more real food meal or drink or snack per week (which I don't think is overwhelming for an individual or a family), within two months you'll be at 14 or 15 out of 35 meals and you will have literally doubled the amount of nutrients you are eating. For many, that would change your life in such a wonderful way. Plus you will now be consuming far fewer potentially problematic substances.

Double the amount of green plant foods you currently eat

- Add a green smoothie for breakfast or for a snack.

- Take nutrient-dense leftovers for lunch instead of buying a sandwich with only a token amount of greens in it.

- Use my cookbooks, *Real Food Chef*, *Real Food Kitchen* and *Sweet Food Story*, to find recipes and guidance that will help you amp up the greens and other plants in your daily diet.

- Follow the digestive system strategies outlined later in this chapter to maximize nourishment (see page 226).

Cut out or significantly limit caffeine

- Take a break from coffee, black tea, and caffeinated soft drinks (soda) for four weeks.

- When you visit your favorite café choose green tea or herbal tea or a dandelion tea (made like a latte), or less often a decaf (make sure it is Swiss water filtered to limit your consumption of the usual chemicals used to decaffeinate coffee beans – most cafés have the Swiss water filtered decaf these days), or order a green juice.

- After eliminating caffeine for four weeks, if you want to bring it back after your four-week break, only drink it when you go out for breakfast or perhaps on the weekends.

- Remember it is what you do every day that impacts your health the most, not what you do occasionally – your rituals create your life.

Cut out or significantly limit alcohol

- Get honest with yourself about how alcohol affects you and those around you.

- If you drink it every day, it stops being special, so drink only on special occasions.

- If you drink every day it is too much.

- If you consume more than 200ml of wine a day and have fewer than two AFDs per week, scientific research suggests you are damaging your health.

- Swap alcohol for sparkling water with fresh lemon or lime.

- If you want to keep drinking, swap wine for a gin or vodka and soda with fresh lemon or lime for four weeks, as this way you will tend to drink less alcohol (one standard drink instead of three per glass), less sugar, no preservatives, which are all liver loaders.

Restorative movement

If you are SNS dominant from the way you live your life, adding more factors to your world that promote SNS dominance will not solve your rush.

Remember, you often resist the most, what you need the most. I witness this in my work with clients every week of my life. If you are currently into loads of cardio, you may tell me that yoga will 'bore you to tears.' I call cardio 'yang' exercise and I describe some forms of yoga as 'yin.' Most rushing women need to incorporate more yin movement into their lifestyle on a regular basis. I also encourage women to do some form of regular resistance training whether that be using weights or simply using their own body weight.

Some form of yin movement needs to be incorporated a minimum of three times into your week. Ideally set up a daily ritual. But if that means starting out with a once-a-week session then that is wonderful. Yin begets yin. If you insist on continuing to cardio it up every day, start your day with a yin movement (see below).

Yin movement includes:

Qi gong

- These slow breathing exercises and gentle movements are a delicious way to start the day.

- Qi gong helps you to cultivate your energy and regular practice can lead to better sleep and more vibrant energy during the day.

Restorative yoga

- Consists of yoga poses, pranayama (extension and control of the breath), breath awareness exercises, and meditation (training the mind in openness and kindness). The technique helps restore the body/mind connection.

- It is particularly beneficial for those who identified with pituitary depletion, adrenal depletion, or thyroid depletion.

- It is outstanding at regulating the menstrual cycle and for fertility.

- Stillness Through Movement is a process where one learns to align with one's true consciousness/intelligence (rather than the stories). Created by Tracy Whitton, it is a true gift for all women, particularly rushing women.

- Through breath and mind awareness you are able to let go deeply allowing you to receive the benefits of the restorative pose, bringing the body/ mind back to its natural state of peace and contentment.

- Without this awareness you tend to live in a permanent state of unease, so when you practice in this way you begin to align with the ease of life. Your new saying might just become 'Life is simple and easy!'

- The parasympathetic nervous system is effectively activated during restorative yoga. As you now know, the PNS is responsible for balancing the body and bringing its response system back into equilibrium. Restorative yoga takes the spine and nervous system out of the flight-or-fight response, relaxing and calming the adrenals.

- To do this props are used to support the body so no strain occurs; yet you can hold any posture anywhere from two to 20 minutes. It is sometimes referred to as 'active relaxation.'

- Some poses target a certain area or gland, such as the pituitary, where others have an overall benefit. All poses create specific physiological responses, which are beneficial to health and can reduce the effects of stress-related disease.

- In general restorative practice is great for those times when one feels weak, fatigued, or stressed from day-to-day activities or for those who find other styles of yoga too difficult.

- These poses are especially beneficial for those times before, during, and after major life transitions like: death of a loved one, change of job, pregnancy, marriage, new baby, children leaving home, divorce, or adrenal burnout. You can also practice the poses when ill, recovering from an illness or injury, or simply as part of your daily or weekly routine.

- It is great for rebalancing hormones in women who have PMS, challenging puberty, menstruation, or menopause.

- What is also exceptional about restorative yoga is it doesn't matter whether you have never experienced yoga before or have been practicing for 30 years. This yoga can guide you to where you need to go. I personally LOVE it.

Meditation

- The stillness that comes from regular meditation is in itself a journey and a reward.

- If your mind is super busy find a CD you like that can guide you. I recommend 'Stillness Through Movement' created by Tracy Whitton; it is the most wonderfully restorative movement I have experienced.

- It can help to have someone talking or asking you to imagine things for a period of time when the meditation first starts. And then once the mind is quieter, you will embody the stillness on offer.

- Remember that meditation takes practice. In the same way you can't run a marathon without any training. You have to work up to the distance with practice runs. The mind is the same. It takes practice to train it.

The following piece was written by one of my clients who resisted meditation initially but stuck with it and reaped the benefits:

Today I had my usual pang of anxiety about the future and getting sick, being in an accident, losing someone who is close to me (my mind is incessant; it never stops), but then something amazing happened. I just let myself fall into the feelings and the whole thing opened up. I had read about this before but never experienced it. I felt like the entire night sky, filled with stars, was inside me. It was really amazing being able to witness a moment of terror and pain transform into something calming and expansive.

• • • • • • • • • • • • • • • • • • •

Restorative sleep

As discussed earlier, there are a few things I link to amazing health. Optimal nutrition, of course, fresh air, movement, love, forgiveness, and great sleep.

Sleep affects our physical and mental health enormously. Sleep is often the only time our PNS can dominate, and I suspect that for many women who don't sleep well, it isn't even happening overnight. It is vital that you schedule maximum sleep time for yourself if you want to start feeling bliss from the inside out. Restorative sleep is critical to every level of our health. Of course, if you have little ones that need you during the night, support yourself to sleep when you can, and remember to breathe and remind yourself that they are little for such a short time.

If you do not sleep well or you do not feel restored after sleep, apply any (or all!) of the strategies below. The overall concept here is to do whatever it takes to get you to stop churning out adrenalin.

Omit caffeine for eight weeks

- Sources of caffeine to avoid include soft drinks and chocolate, as well as the obvious sources of tea and coffee.

- Wean off caffeine, if you currently have more than two caffeinated drinks per day, by having a green tea daily for three days and then omitting completely.

- After eight weeks, if it has helped, choose whether you return to including caffeine in your day and, if you do, take care to include it only a couple of times a week.

Omit alcohol

- You may feel like it helps you fall asleep but it tends to disturb sleep patterns during the night as it prevents you from going into the restorative, deep REM sleep.

Practice good sleep hygiene

- Do not sit in bright light for two hours before you want to go to bed.

- Get up at the same time each morning and expose your eyes to sunlight. Light destroys your sleep hormone melatonin and allows your happy, calm, content hormone called serotonin to surge.

- Avoid doing work for a minimum of two hours before bed and engaging your brain in this way.

- Consider the age of your mattress: Dust, mold, and sweat all accumulate in mattresses plus beds lose their support. You spend one-third of your life in bed so it is best to make it a place that brings out an 'ahhh' moment of bliss when you fall into it each night. This 'ahhh' moment alone is good for your health!

- If your mattress is more than 10 years old, it is most likely not supporting you well and the waste accumulation may be affecting your health. This is particularly true if you experience allergies to dust, mold, and/or have asthma.

Schedule some daily calm

- Schedule (and do!) 20 long slow deep breaths daily.

- Do restorative yoga poses daily.

- Meditate and/or pray regularly.

Restorative actions

Remember to feel your feelings because part of growing up is learning that your feelings will not destroy you. They are just feelings. And they too shall pass.

And when you are grateful you cannot be stressed, so make gratitude a daily practice. Say out loud or write down each day at least three things which you are grateful for. If you don't know where to start, just think about the simple things in life, such as nature or breathing in fresh air or the smile on a loved one's face. If you haven't already, you might want to start a journal to capture your gratitude and any other murmurings that bubble to the surface while you are in this space. Insight often comes this way and we get clarity about something that perhaps we felt confused about.

Feeling like your life has purpose and meaning is crucial to restorative actions. Contribution is key here. When you make a difference in someone else's life, your heart feels fulfilled. As the poet Rabindranath Tagore so beautifully said: 'I slept and dreamt that life was joy. I awoke and saw that life was service. I acted and behold, service was joy.'

- Pick up any litter you see.

- Call people you may not have caught up with for ages – they will be thrilled.

- Volunteer for a cause close to your heart or a local community project.

  A male friend of mine who works in more than a full-time job was standing on a street corner collecting money for the City Mission. Among many things, they raise money for food to feed people on Christmas Day. My friend said he does a half-day for them every month and I had no idea. He'd never mentioned it. He said it was the least he could do because he has so much.

  . . . .

- Bake a cake and deliver it to an aged care facility and stay a while and talk to the residents; you will make their day and you will learn something.

- Give away clothes and household goods you no longer need to an organization that can use them.

- Smile while you walk along the street.

- Notice the color of the sky wherever you are.

- Send someone a card in the mail to let them know you are thinking of them.

  My amazing mum has sent me an envelope packed with bits and pieces every week of my life since I left home to wherever I am in the world! It is usually filled with pictures from magazines she has collected that she thinks I will like and the births, deaths, and marriages from the local paper from my hometown. It always makes my day. Thanks Mum.

  . . . .

- If you think of something that amuses you and you think it would entertain someone else, tell them, text them, and share the giggles.

- If you see someone looking lost ask them if you can help.

- Practice random acts of kindness.

- Be kind. As I love to say, kindness must come first.

We are all connected

Something very special unfolds in our lives when we remember that we are part of a universe that connects all things. For when we recall that, it often fosters a desire to contribute to the world beyond our own immediate gain. I find the happiest and healthiest people are often those making a difference to what I have come to call 'the greater good' in ways that are meaningful to them. When we turn up to a job each day that we don't really like and that is jam-packed with pressure, yet our perception is that to be responsible we must stay there, I find that engaging in activities that are meaningful to you somehow eases the pain, pressure, and exhaustion of that work, especially if the work is not meaningful to you.

> I once met a rushing woman who was beyond stressed. And when I asked her why she told me it was because she had 23 Christmas presents to buy before Christmas and it was already November 24. I thought she must have had an overwhelming number of other commitments between now and Christmas but she said she didn't. No work, nothing major scheduled, no major family dramas. Without judgment, I gently suggested to my client that she needed a reality check and asked if she had ever considered how blessed she was firstly to have 23 people to buy for and secondly to have the financial means to pay for these gifts. I watched her face respond like a typical rushing woman with expressions of

guilt and realized that sometimes we get so caught up with ourselves that we forget we are part of a greater whole.

• • • • • • • • • • • • • • • • • • •

I've also met countless people who have quit financially rewarding jobs to spend a year or the rest of the foreseeable future doing something that is more meaningful to them. Do something you care about. Sometimes sadness crops up in an attempt to wake you up to your passion. I am not suggesting for one second that you quit your job. I'm simply suggesting you find a way to contribute to the world around you and witness a part of you wake up to the joy that has always been there.

Radiant living

There are many different forms of yoga and yoga means different things to different people. I find people gravitate to yoga for a wide variety of reasons. For some it is movement. For some it is a path to stillness. Some begin because they developed a degenerative disease such as cancer. For others it is just a cool thing to do; all of their friends are doing it. For others it is a preventative health practice and for others it is part of their spiritual journey. For many it is how they bring balance into their very hectic lives. In yoga circles they talk of the Sages' 10 Rituals of Radiant Living. I encourage you to embrace them in ways that are meaningful to you.

- Ritual of Solitude

- Ritual of Physicality

- Ritual of Nourishment

- Ritual of Abundant Knowledge

- Ritual of Personal Reflection

- Ritual of Early Awakening

- Ritual of Music

- Ritual of Spoken Word

- Ritual of Congruent Character

- Ritual of Simplicity

Keep a journal

Buy yourself a beautiful notebook that can be your journal. Capture anything you like in there. Be sure to express your gratitude as a daily ritual. If you feel like you don't have time, keep it in the living room or the kitchen... some place in your house where you will see it. Keep a pen with it or, better still, some colored markers and whenever you clap eyes on it, think of something for which you are grateful and write it down!

Stop, keep, start

Another great thing to do with a journal is to make a three-column list with the following headings: 'Stop,' 'Keep,' and 'Start'.

Fill each column in as you think of things by answering the questions:

- What am I going to stop doing?

- What am I going to keep doing?

- What am I going to start doing?

Stop, keep, and start goals can make change fun, manageable, and suitable for your lifestyle. Use the following suggestion to give you ideas. Here is a sample:

Stop: I'm going to stop getting caught up in gossip as it's exhausting.

Keep: I'm going to keep eating a nourishing breakfast every day.

Start: I'm going to start walking four days out of seven for the next two weeks starting tomorrow morning at 6:00am.

Exploring your inner world and emotional landscape

The peace you seek is within you. To help you explore your inner world, to begin inquiry, to help you understand your subconscious reactions more, to help you lose the emotional charge from a relationship that in your head you are over, but yet your body still seems to react to.

Try any of the following:

NSA (Network Spinal Analysis)

- NSA involves gentle precise touch to the spine, which cues the brain to create new wellness-promoting strategies.

- Two unique healing waves develop with this work. They are associated with spontaneous release of spinal and life tensions, and the use of existing tension as fuel for spinal reorganization and enhanced wellness.

- Practitioners combine their clinical assessments of spinal refinements with a patient's self-assessments of wellness and life changes.

- Greater self-awareness and conscious awakening of the relationships between the body, mind, emotion, and expression of the human spirit are realized through this popular healing work.

- NSA is exclusively practiced by chiropractors.

The Journey

- Created by Brandon Bays, this process (described in her book of the same name) allows you to 'see' the world as it really is, rather than the stories you have constructed around things.

- This process allows you to see the beliefs that no longer serve you and allows them to fall away effortlessly. And as you now understand when your beliefs change, your behavior changes, as your behaviors are the outermost expression of your beliefs.

- The Journey is a powerful healing tool through simply fostering the innate healing within you.

It would not surprise me if, one day, science shows what many people already believe to be true – that cellular changes can be fostered through thought. I truly believe this to be the case.

The work of Tony Robbins

- Tony's book *Awaken the Giant Within* is brilliant. Don't just read it... do the exercises in it!

- Attend one of Tony's live events, such as Date With Destiny, as these are powerful beyond measure. He is a genius.

- Tony Robbins's work (also available on CD) can help you to see and then change any limiting beliefs, and avoid negative emotions and foster those you want to experience.

- His work, his contribution to the world, has forever changed the face of psychology and helps people, no matter how massive or relatively small their past hurts may have been, move forward into an empowered future.

Restorative yoga

I discussed the benefits of restorative yoga earlier in this chapter (see page 202). I personally had never experienced such deep stillness before restorative yoga became part of my life. The gracious, kind, and insightful Tracy Whitton was my first teacher of this beautiful practice, and I am eternally grateful to her for developing what she has come to call 'Stillness Through Movement.' Thank you for sharing this with the world, beautiful lady.

The Serenity Prayer

Don't worry about something until it's a problem. If it becomes a problem, then you can face it, but worrying about something that truly may never happen only serves to hurt you. As we now know, stress, whether it is real or perceived, may promote the production of excess cortisol and drive SNS dominance. The ripple effect of a worry can very slowly and subtly change your mood and your metabolism. And it's the chemical signals of your body that are driving this. The beautiful, old piece of wisdom called 'The Serenity Prayer' is useful to remember and act on, especially if you are a worrier:

> *'Grant me the serenity to accept the things I cannot change,*
> *Courage to change the things I can,*
> *And the wisdom to know the difference.'*

And as Geneen Roth so eloquently says, 'Every time you stop fighting with the way things are, you return to yourself, to heaven on earth. Can you stop fighting today? Can you give yourself that much of heaven?'

There is great freedom and a slice of heaven in acceptance (which is not the same as complacency).

Useful tests to explore your biochemistry

To examine your 'rushing' biochemistry, to explore your hormone levels thoroughly, you can visit a health professional and have your blood and/or saliva tested. Useful blood tests include:

Thyroid group

- TSH

- T3

- Reverse T3

- T4

- Antithyroid peroxidase antibodies (anti-TPO)

- Antithyroglobulin (anti-TG)

Adrenal

- Cortisol: urinary 24-hour collection or first morning collection

Ovarian (some are also related to pituitary function)

- Estrogen

- Progesterone

- LH

- FSH

Vitamin D

- Many people are deficient in this crucial nutrient. Have yours tested and supplement if it is low. It is involved in countless vital processes in your body.

Cholesterol
....

- This is the building block of your steroid hormones and elevated levels indicate that the liver needs support (see also liver support strategies below).

If your results come back out of the 'normal' range or skewed one way, strategies are offered below for each of the groups above (for cholesterol employ the liver support strategies). It can be very useful to seek guidance from a health professional to guide you specifically. If your blood tests come back 'normal' yet you exhibit all of the symptoms for dysfunction with a particular gland, find someone who will work with you to treat your symptoms rather than your blood work. I have clients all over the world who fall into this category.

The body gives us symptoms to communicate that it wants us to live differently – perhaps eat differently or think differently. I believe in every moment we are given a second chance.

Strategies to assist your body systems

As you were reading each chapter, there may have been body systems that jumped out at you, resonating with what you are experiencing. This section is designed to guide you with solutions or considerations for the systems that you know need support. Remember, nothing in the body stands alone, which is why a holistic approach is vital.

Nervous system

The whole goal of this book as well as the following strategies is to assist you to spend far more time in your daily life with your parasympathetic nervous system being dominant or certainly to allow the two arms of your nervous system to be balanced and respond appropriately, rather than the SNS always running the show, for in this latter scenario, our health on every level is compromised.

General solutions:

- The way you breathe is key, even though that sounds too simple to make a difference.

- Start the day with 20 long slow breaths before you get out of bed or, alternatively, breathe and move your diaphragm while you wait for the kettle to boil, or while you sit at traffic lights.

- Enroll in a breath-focused movement class two to four times a week, such as tai chi, qi gong, or restorative yoga (see page 202).

- Start the day with yin movement (see page 202), followed by an egg-based breakfast for two weeks, and notice if this sets your day up better.

- Swap coffee for green tea (except if you have problems with sleep, see also Chapter 2, page 28), and notice if you feel calmer and more energized an hour later after a week of doing this.

- Add more fat to your meals, particularly lunch, in the form of avocado, nuts, organic butter, tahini, oily fish, and observe if your desire for sweet food mid-afternoon diminishes. That way you can choose a healthy afternoon tea, rather than be ruled by that 'eat your arm off' feeling.

Emotional support

If you recognize that you do tend to try to be all things to all people or perhaps you walk on eggshells around a boss or a family member who at times has an explosive temper... consider seeking the assistance of a health professional with this and learn how to change the way you approach these situations. The patterns mostly get set up in childhood. My suggestions include:

- Consulting with an NSA (network spinal analysis) practitioner.

- Going on a 'Date With Destiny' (www.tonyrobbins.com) or reading *Awaken the Giant Within* by Tony Robbins (see also page 213).

- Attending a 'Beautiful You Weekend' that I run for women.

- Doing the online 'Rushing Woman's Syndrome Quickstart Course,' which I created to support this book.

- Seeing a psychologist.

- Seeing an NLP (neuro-linguistic programming) practitioner.

- Seeing an EFT (emotional freedom technique) practitioner.

Adrenals

How high your level of stress is and how you feel your body copes with it will influence the steps you take. The above section of solutions is general, and I can confidently say that virtually everyone will benefit from applying them.

The herbs used for adrenal support are beautiful, however it is best to check with a qualified medical herbalist to find out about herbs that will meet your specific needs. I have made comments beside most of the herbs about their applications.

If you have identified that you are adrenally fatigued and beyond exhausted on a daily basis, see also adrenal fatigue supplementation below and consider including a restorative yoga practice (see page 202). General solutions for adrenal support include:

- Schedule and commit to regular breathing exercises. It can literally change your life. And I do not say that lightly.

- Practice Stillness Through Movement, yoga, Pilates, tai chi, or qi gong a minimum of twice a week for four weeks. Develop a daily practice for outstanding results.

- Spend five minutes daily focusing on and giving voice to all the aspects of your life for which you are grateful; you can't be stressed when you feel grateful.

Supplements

- With the guidance of a herbalist, take some adrenal support herbs. Not all herbal medicine is created equal, however, so you want to ensure the brand you take is reputable. Check that it has been tested by a high-level quality control system and that the active ingredients said to be in the product are indeed present, as well as no contaminants. Herbal medicine can be taken in a liquid tincture form or as tablets. The majority of the following adrenal herbs are adaptogens, meaning they help the body adapt to stress by fine-tuning the stress response. They include:

- Withania for the worriers

- Rhodiola for the drama queens or occasionally for the worriers

- Siberian ginseng for the fatigued feminine

- Panex ginseng for the utterly fatigued

- Licorice, especially if your blood pressure is on the low end of normal

- Dandelion leaves, especially if you retain fluid

- The adrenals also love vitamins B and C, and for adrenal

support I usually supplement both. I am a fan of food-based nutritional supplements.

Just as important, if not the most important aspect of supporting adrenal function for a balanced and appropriate stress hormone response, is the application of the emotional health strategies (see Chapter 9, page 157) and diaphragmatic breathing (see Chapter 4, page 65).

Adrenal fatigue supplementation

As I outlined in the adrenal chapter for people with deep, deep fatigue, I almost always use the following herbal tonic that contains:

- Panex ginseng
- Licorice
- Dandelion leaves
- Astragalus
- One other herb depending on what else is going on for the individual (a liver herb or a reproductive herb are typical)

The restorative power of real food

- Although I often recommend good-quality supplements of herbs and/or nutrients for adrenal fatigue (and other health conditions), never underestimate the healing and restorative power of food the way it comes in nature (see page 199).

- Taking supplements is not a reason to eat a poor-quality, low-nutrient diet. I simply recommend high-quality supplements where appropriate and particularly to assist in the restoration of health.

Sex hormone balance

Resolving a sex hormone imbalance can change the quality of your life dramatically. Here are some roads for you to consider.

PMS and menstrual cycle challenges

- If you have any type of menstrual cycle or reproductive system challenges, take a four-week break from alcohol or, better still, take a break from it for two menstrual cycles.

- PMS typically significantly decreases without alcohol, as the liver is more efficiently able to clear estrogen from the body (see Chapter 5, page 81).

- If this solution is 'impossible,' decrease alcohol intake to two nights a week, and drink less than half a bottle of wine.

- Coffee can be another big-ticket item when it comes to PMS. Consider swapping coffee for green tea for four weeks, or preferably two menstrual cycles, and see how you feel (see Chapter 5, page 83).

- Take a four-week strict break from all dairy products. Better still; omit them for two menstrual cycles.

For PMS, it is important to know what is creating the PMS: is it too much estrogen in the second half of the cycle? If so, the liver needs support. Is it caused by low progesterone due to the constant, relentless output of stress hormones (telling the body it is not 'safe' to have a baby at the moment)? If so, the adrenals and nervous system needs support. Or is both liver and adrenal support necessary? The latter is a very common scenario these days particularly among rushing women. Or are you not ovulating, leading to no progesterone? If so, this needs correcting, which usually requires improving the relationship between the pituitary and the ovaries. How are these things achieved?

For estrogen dominance (second half of cycle)

- Extracts of broccoli or broccoli sprouts. I am all for getting what we need from our food, but, in this case, you need to eat eight heads of broccoli a day to get the same therapeutic effect as one good-quality capsule of broccoli extract. You'll find it in my Bio Blends range of food-based nutritional supplements.

For estrogen dominance due to the liver recycling estrogen

- Apply the liver support strategies listed elsewhere (see page 230).

- Decrease liver loaders.

- Support the liver detoxification biochemical pathways by eating whole real foods, especially plants.

- Consider using a food-based nutritional liver support that contains herbs/plants such as:

  ~ St. Mary's thistle

  ~ Globe artichoke

  ~ Turmeric

  ~ Gentian

  ~ Broccoli

- Eat more bitter foods; most green vegetables have a bitter taste base.

I designed my food-based nutritional supplements to support people safely and effectively. Visit www.bioblends.co.nz for more information about products such as Liver Love, Cycle Essentials and Sleep Restore.

For low progesterone due to elevated stress hormones

- Focus on the adrenal and nervous system support strategies (see page 261 onwards).

- Regular, breath-focused practices are essential (see Chapter 4, page 65 onwards).

- For herbs specific to the stress response refer to the adrenal and nervous system solutions sections (see pages 219–220).

- Herbs and nutrients that are specifically useful for balancing estrogen to progesterone through a variety of mechanisms include:

    ~ Licorice

    ~ Peonia

    ~ Iodine

    ~ Selenium

    ~ Vitamin D

Menopause strategies

- For hot flashes consider whether the heat is coming from low estrogen, liver/gallbladder congestion, or both?

- For low estrogen:

    ~ Black cohosh

    ~ Sage

- For the liver/gallbladder

    ~ Globe artichoke

- ~ St. Mary's thistle
- ~ Dandelion
- ~ Turmeric
- ~ Bupleurum
- ~ Schisandra
- For adrenal support
  - ~ Rhodiola, if you are also exhausted
  - ~ Siberian ginseng
  - ~ Withania
- For low blood pressure along with stress:
  - ~ Licorice
  - ~ Magnesium

Peri- and postmenopause

As I said earlier in the book, if you are peri- or postmenopausal, I can't encourage you enough to address adrenal health and liver health for these two systems, as well as the overall balance of your nervous system. This tends to make a significant difference to menopause symptoms.

For all the challenges discussed in this chapter, focus on the gifts of your feminine essence (see Chapter 5, page 91).

Thyroid support

See a health professional to be guided about what minerals will be best suited to meet your individual needs. If you have a diagnosed, underactive thyroid condition and you are on synthetic medication but your symptoms are still present, explore transitioning to whole thyroid extract under medical supervision. Or you may need additional iodine, selenium, iron and/or essential fats.

More general suggestions:

- Go on a grain-free diet trial for a minimum of four weeks.

- If you love dairy products and the idea of going without cheese makes you wonder if you could, then do it! Remember, it is often what we love (not just like) to eat that can be a problem. Do a four-week dairy-free trial if this is the case.

- Support liver and gallbladder function to assist with bowel elimination. Globe artichoke is particularly good for 'thyroid' people.

- Refer to the advice about estrogen dominance (see page 222).

- Adrenal support is almost essential, especially when beginning to treat the thyroid. Refer to the stress hormones chapter and also refresh on adrenal support strategies (see page 218).

- You will probably crave coffee. Please explore taking a four-week break and observe how you feel at the end of this period. Use green tea, which has a low caffeine level, instead (see Chapter 2, page 28).

- Explore how you can change the 'demands' on your time if you have an overactive thyroid by revising the thyroid and emotions chapters (see Chapters 6 and 9, pages 103 and 157).

Pituitary Support

When the pituitary is at the heart of your problems (please understand I am not referring to pituitary diseases), you will often have suboptimal health with a number of endocrine organs, which may include the ovaries (sex hormones), the adrenals (stress hormones), and/or the thyroid (thyroid hormones).

When I suspect the pituitary needs some support I will tend to use Vitex in a woman who is menstruating and Rhodiola postmenopausally.

Women with a pituitary that is not functioning optimally due to too much SNS dominance will often feel better addressing adrenal, ovarian, and thyroid function. Pick one and start there. Or simply start with the pituitary enhancing Stillness Through Movement.

Other general suggestions:

- Restorative yoga
- Herbs
  - ~ Vitex
  - ~ Alfalfa
  - ~ Ginseng family
  - ~ Licorice
- Sandalwood or clary sage oil massaged into soles of feet and/or reproductive organ areas

Digestion support

Digestion is central and essential to every process in our body. It is the base on which we build. So, whether your aim is to slow down, weigh less, optimize your health and wellbeing, and/or improve a challenging or diseased gut, or all of the above, understanding your digestive system is a crucial step to optimal health.

Remember the key ingredients to good digestion:

- Slow down! Chew your food.

- Eat in a calm state.

- Look at the food while you eat it. Do not read or watch TV.

- Include fats and/or protein with each meal as you are likely to eat less and be satisfied with less total food for that meal, than if you simply eat carbohydrates on their own.

- Eat less. Reduce your portion size by one quarter, especially in the evening if you overeat, and see how you feel.

- Wake your stomach acid up before you eat by using lemon juice in warm water or apple cider vinegar before meals, breakfast in particular.

- Drink water between meals, not with them.

- If efficient bowel evacuation is a particular challenge for you, reference *Accidentally Overweight* and the numerous strategies outlined there.

- Omit a food you feel you cannot live without for a trial period of four weeks. The first four to seven days will be the most difficult but persevere. The results may be enormously worth it.

- Working with a wonderful practitioner of Traditional Chinese Medicine can also assist you in healing your gut.

- Try aloe vera juice to start your day if you have a particularly irritated gut.

- Use an organic green drink made of powdered vegetables.

- If you suspect a parasite infection, the herbs black walnut and Chinese wormwood are excellent, as is oregano oil.

Gut bacteria

- Apply all of the above strategies first to see if that helps. Often the bad guys have been able to take over because of the pH of the large intestine and this is mostly influenced by what goes on higher up in the digestive system.

- If these strategies don't work, trial a probiotic supplement that is only Bifidobacterium species.

Food intolerance or reaction (if you suspect you are reacting adversely to a food)

- Omit the suspected food from your diet for a period of four weeks.

- If it makes no difference, bring it back. If it helps, leave it out for three months and then try it again. Or if you are happy to go without it, then do so.

- If it is a food that is a rich source of nutrients, for example, gluten-containing foods tend to be a good source of B vitamins, then you will need to supplement.

- It may also be necessary to use a mineral supplement that contains a combination of calcium, magnesium, manganese, boron, and vitamin D if you omit dairy products.

- This is of lesser importance if your diet is plant-based and highly alkaline. It is best to seek the guidance of a health professional with this last point and particularly if you are going to omit food/s to get a resolution of your symptoms.

Colonics

Another remedy that many people have strong opinions about is colon hydrotherapy or 'colonics,' as they are known. This process involves a tube being inserted into the rectum through which warm or cool water gently flows. It allows the hardened fecal matter to soften causing the large bowel to empty fully, getting rid of built-up waste that may have been there for a very long time. I have had clients tell me that the waste they excreted during their first colonic was black, implying that it may have been there for many years and interfering with healthy bowel function. One lady told me she saw popcorn in the 'viewing' pipe during her colonic and she knew that the last time she ate popcorn was when she'd been to the movies – six months ago!

Colonics polarize people. The idea either appeals or it doesn't. There is no middle ground, and they seem to serve some people and upset the balance in others. But don't lose sight of what trends have done to medicine. Up until the early 1900s, colon hydrotherapy was part of general medicine, and doctors understood the importance of good bowel evacuation. In fact, coffee enemas were actually cited in the *Merck Manual for Doctors* for liver detoxification until 1972. It is a very personal choice.

When you examine the history of medicine and observe the split between what we now know to be Western medicine and complementary medicine, it is clear why this happened; however, this book does not seek to explore this segregation in detail. I will simply say that colonics were once accepted as a very 'normal' treatment method for a host of health conditions, not just bowel issues. With a well-functioning bowel, an enormous load is not only taken off the digestive system but also the liver, the organ primarily responsible for cleaning the body.

Help prevent bowel cancer by ensuring efficient bowel evacuation using methods that suit you! Always seek advice from a health professional before undertaking colon hydrotherapy if it appeals to you.

Liver supports

If you identify that your liver health needs to be addressed to assist you stop rushing and reacting with anger, here are some solutions for your liver:

Omitting and/or reducing alcohol and caffeine

- Make time-based goals. For example, 'I will only drink alcohol on weekends for four weeks,' or 'I will only drink coffee when I go out for breakfast on Sundays.'

- Take a break from alcohol.

- Only drink on weekends; no alcohol during the week.

- Replace coffee with green or white tea (or, less often, weak, black tea).

Herbal and nutritional support options

- St. Mary's thistle, especially if alcohol is a regular part of your life.

- Globe artichoke, especially if you have a tendency to constipation and/or a liver roll (fat roll under your bra), and/or central torso tenderness.

- Turmeric, particularly if you consume many liver loaders and experience inflammation.

- Bupleurum, especially if there are clots in your menstrual blood.

- Schisandra, especially for its detox action (it also works on the adrenals).

- Transform anger into passion by giving a different meaning to a past experience; the energy of anger and passion are the same.

- Drink vegetable juice or a 'green smoothie' each morning or use an organic green powder.

- Snack on seeds and nuts.

- Eat less fruit and none after your morning tea.

- Cut out dairy products for a four-week trial and/or cut out grains (containing gluten) for a four-week trial.

- Take an essential fatty acid supplement, such as a good-quality, decent dose of fish oil for reducing cholesterol, or a flax oil and evening primrose combination.

- Eat high zinc foods, such as oysters (from clean waters) or take a daily zinc supplement of 15–30mg zinc picolinate – best taken at night just before bed to maximize absorption.

Remember, it is what you do every day that impacts your health, not what you do occasionally. Just get honest with yourself. And take such good care of yourself that your quality of life is forever excellent. We only have one liver!

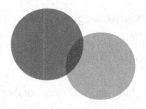

The Wrap-Up

M y favorite quote spoken by His Holiness the Dalai Lama is
this:

> 'When asked "What thing about humanity surprises you the
> most?" the Dalai Lama answered: "Man... because he sacrifices
> his health in order to make money. Then he sacrifices money
> to recuperate his health. And then he is so anxious about the
> future that he does not enjoy the present; the result being that
> he does not live in the present or the future; he lives as if he is
> never going to die, and then dies having never really lived."'

And it breaks my heart that this is true for so many people. I want
you to live in love and from love, not in fear. It is crucial 'you'
don't disappear. The world needs you. And for you to be happy,
for you to feel the joy, for you to be able to appreciate the many,
many magical moments on offer to you, you so desperately need
to slow down.

So, as I said I would, I've given you information, solutions, and
strategies to begin this wonderful process from rush to rest. We have
explored bringing calm and spaciousness back into life. Consider
with kindness and curiosity, rather than judgment, what has led you
to sacrifice your own needs and potentially your optimal health and

pursue whatever it was you thought you wanted – which remember is almost always the means to gain the love and approval of someone significant to you.

And once you've caught even a glimpse of that – of what has been driving you – your life will never be the same again. You may still get caught in the rush sometimes, but you won't get stuck there and you certainly won't sacrifice your health. You'll find you have more of a voice, if you have been more of a 'keep the peace' kind of female, because there has been a shift in your level of self-care and how far you will go to preserve that. Plus by always doing things for others, they'll never experience what it is like to give to you or get the opportunity to grow.

But if you do get caught in the rush, you'll notice much sooner and you'll giggle and I hope you find it fun to explore what led you there that time. There is so much joy and beauty when you follow anything to its end.

I wish I could tell you that if the idea of applying strategies to combat your rush and the health consequences of your rush is not for you, then you could simply 'do' the most feminine of 'solutions'... and that is to simply be... I wish I could tell you that worked. But right now, if you are juggling a million things and there are still a million unattended to, 'being' ain't going to just happen. If all of the above feel overwhelming to you and like just another to-do list that you will never ever have all ticked off, then simply begin with two things: your long, slow diaphragmatic breaths and taking a break from caffeine. Commit to these daily for four weeks. Begin there.

And while you're at it, become so aware of what you say to yourself. Become aware of when you say cruel things to yourself and catch yourself. Work out what led you there. It will almost always be a feeling that you are not (good) enough and therefore won't be loved. When you see that's all it was and as an adult you are 'safe' – and those feelings and thoughts are nothing but an old outdated story you've been telling yourself – you'll find that a little piece of you that's been asleep will wake up. And let that piece of you be the part that takes such good care of you for the world needs you... needs you happy and healthy to share your gifts with it! May you have a healthy body, an open heart, and a peaceful mind.

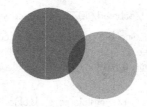

References

1. www.cancer.org.au/policy-and-advocacy/position-statements/alcohol-and-cancer/; accessed March 7, 2017

2. www.cancer.gov/about-cancer/causes-prevention/risk/alcohol/alcohol-fact-sheet; accessed March 7, 2017

3. www.cancerresearchuk.org/about-cancer/causes-of-cancer/alcohol-and-cancer/how-alcohol-causes-cancer; accessed March 7, 2017

4. www.breastcancer.org/risk/factors/alcohol; accessed March 7, 2017

5. Smith-Warner, S.A., et al. 'Alcohol and Breast Cancer in Women: A Pooled Analysis of Cohort Studies,' JAMA, 1998; 279(7): 535–40; doi: 10.1001/jama.279.7.535

6. www.nhs.uk/news/2015/08August/Pages/Just-one-drink-a-day-may-raise-breast-cancer-risk.aspx; accessed March 7, 2017

7. Min-Jing, et al., 'Green tea compounds in breast cancer prevention and treatment,' World J Clin Oncol. Aug 10, 2014; 5(3): 520–8; doi: 10.5306/wjco.v5.i3.520

8. www.womensinternational.com/connections/breast.html; accessed March 7, 2017

9. www.berkeleywellness.com/healthy-eating/nutrition/article/diet-and-breast-cancer-update; accessed March 7, 2017

10. www.progressreport.cancer.gov/prevention/red_meat; accessed March 7, 2017

11. www.progressreport.cancer.gov/prevention/fat_consumption; accessed March 7, 2017

12. www.cancer.gov/about-cancer/causes-prevention/risk/diet/cruciferous-vegetables-fact-sheet

13. www.ncbi.nlm.nih.gov/pubmed/10736624; accessed March 7, 2017

14. Rock, C. *et al.*, 'Longitudinal biological exposure to carotenoids is associated with breast cancer-free survival in the women's healthy eating and living study,' Cancer Epidemiology, Biomarkers & Prevention, 2009; 18(2): 486–94

15. Kessler, J. 'The effect of supraphysiologic levels of iodine on patients with cyclic mastalgia,' *The Breast Journal*, 2004; 10(4): 328–36

16. Ghent, W. *et al.*, 'Iodine replacement in fibrocystic disease of the breast,' *Canadian Journal of Surgery*, Oct 1993; 35(5): 453–60

17. Eskin, B. *et al.*, 'Mammary Gland dysplasia in iodine deficiency,' JAMA, 1967; 200:115–19

18. health.usnews.com/health-news/health-wellness/articles/2015/04/17/why-kids-are-hitting-puberty-earlier-than-ever; accessed March 7, 2017

19. www.scientificamerican.com/article/early-puberty-causes-and-effects/; accessed March 7, 2017

20. www.psychologytoday.com/articles/199801/the-call-solitude; accessed March 7, 2017

21. www.cancer.org/cancer/cancer-causes/diet-physical-activity/alcohol-use-and-cancer.html

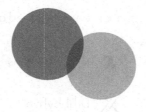

Next Steps

Here is a list of further information that may assist you on your journey. There are books and articles I've cited in the text and listed in the Select Bibliography, if further reading in a particular area interests you.

Nutrition information is always changing and I am passionate about keeping you up to date with the latest and most insightful aspects of health and wellbeing. After reading *Rushing Woman's Syndrome*, you may ask, what's next? I have had many e-mails from people all over the world saying they feel like I've read their diary when it comes to describing how they feel in the pages of this book. People tell me they want more of this type of information and a specific program to follow that encompasses guidance with food, hormone balancing, and strategies that give them further insight into their emotional eating patterns. I cannot encourage you enough to check out the array of options on my website www.drlibby.com where you'll also find the online courses I've created – specifically the Rushing Woman's Syndrome Quickstart Course.

My mission is to educate and inspire people and help them change the relationship they have with their bodies and their health and put the power of choice back in their hands.

I also post health information on social media. Connect with me there at:

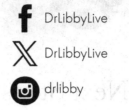

f DrLibbyLive

X DrLibbyLive

⊙ drlibby

And my food-based nutritional supplement range is available from www.bioblends.co.nz

It is an honor to assist you.

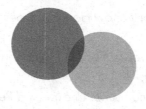

Select Bibliography

Not all of the areas presented in this book have additional resources listed below, as I have read and studied widely (sometimes from very geeky biochemistry textbooks), and this book is the culmination of my knowledge, experience, observation, and intuition in this area to date.

Bennett, Jane and Pope, Alexandra, *The Pill: Are You Sure It's For You?* (Sydney: Allen & Unwin, 2008)

Coates, Dr. Karen and Perry, Vincent, *Embracing the Warrior: An Essential Guide for Women* (Burleigh Heads: Arteriol Press, 2007)

DeVrye, Catherine: www.greatmotivation.com

Epstein, Donny, *The 12 Stages of Healing*, (Amber-Allen Publishers, 1994)

Fasano, Dr. Alessio, *et al.* (2000) 'Zonulin, a newly discovered modulator of intestinal permeability, and its expression in celiac disease,' *The Lancet*, 355; (9214): 1518–1519

Hay, Louise, *You Can Heal Your Life* (Carlsbad: Hay House Inc., 2004)

Northrup, Dr. Christiane, *Women's Bodies Women's Wisdom* (London: Judy Piatkus Ltd, 1998)

Northrup, Kate: www.katenorthrup.com

Pearson, Allison, *I Don't Know How She Does It* (New York: Anchor, 2011)

Robbins, Anthony, *Awaken the Giant Within* (London: Simon & Schuster Ltd, 1992).

Roth, Geneen, *Lost and Found: Unexpected Revelations About Food and Money* (New York: Viking Penguin, 2011)

Weaver, Dr. Libby, *Accidentally Overweight* (Auckland: Little Green Frog, 2011; new edition London: Hay House, 2016)

————, *Rushing Woman's Syndrome* (Auckland: Little Green Frog, 2011)

————, *Beauty from the Inside Out* (Auckland: Little Green Frog, 2013)

————, *The Calorie Fallacy* (Auckland: Little Green Frog, 2014)

————, *Exhausted to Energized* (Auckland: Little Green Frog, 2015)

————, *Women's Wellness Wisdom* (Auckland: Little Green Frog, 2016)

Weaver, Dr. Libby and Tait, Cynthia, *Dr. Libby's Real Food Chef* (Auckland: Little Green Frog, 2012)

————, *Dr. Libby's Real Food Kitchen* (Auckland: Little Green Frog, 2014)

————, *Dr. Libby's Sweet Food Story* (Auckland: Little Green Frog, 2014)

Whitton, Tracy, *Stillness Through Movement* (Gold Coast: Tracy Whitton, 2011)

————, *One With Life CD* (Gold Coast: Tracy Whitton, 2011)

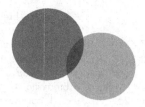

Index

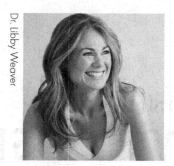

Dr. Libby Weaver

About the Author

Dr. Libby Weaver (PhD) is one of Australasia's leading nutritional biochemists, an author, a speaker, and founder of the food-based supplement range, Bio Blends.

Armed with an abundance of knowledge, scientific research, and a true desire to help people regain their energy and vitality, Dr. Libby empowers and inspires people to take charge of their health and happiness through her books, live events, and nutritional support range.

Having sold over 300,000 books across New Zealand and Australia, she is a nine-times number one bestselling author.

A respected international speaker, Dr. Libby's expertise in nutritional biochemistry has led her to share the stage with Marianne Williamson, Sir Richard Branson, Tony Robbins and Dr. Oz. She is regularly called on as an authoritative figure in the health and wellness industry and has been featured in numerous media publications including *The Times, The Huffington Post, Sydney Morning Herald,* and *The Australian Women's Weekly.* She also appears regularly on breakfast radio and television.

With a natural ability to break even the most complex of concepts into layman's terms, Dr. Libby's health messages embrace her unique three-pillared approach that explores the interplay between nutrition, emotions, and the biochemistry of the body.

It's no surprise that Hollywood husband and wife Hugh Jackman and Deborra-Lee Furness describe her as a "one stop shop in achieving and maintaining ultimate health and wellbeing."

www.drlibby.com

CONNECT WITH

HAY HOUSE
ONLINE

 hayhouse.co.uk   **f** @hayhouse

 @hayhouseuk   **X** @hayhouseuk

 @hayhouseuk   @hayhouseuk

Find out all about our latest books & card decks • Be the first to know about exclusive discounts • Interact with our authors in live broadcasts • Celebrate the cycle of the seasons with us • Watch free videos from your favourite authors • Connect with like-minded souls

'*The gateways to wisdom and knowledge are always open.*'

Louise Hay